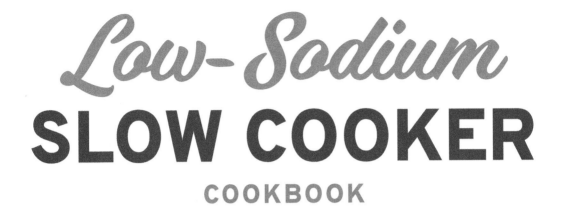

Low-Sodium SLOW COOKER

COOKBOOK

Over 100 Heart-Healthy Recipes That Prep Fast and Cook Slow

Shannon Epstein

Photography by
MARIJA VIDAL

T0020728

R
ROCKRIDGE
PRESS

Copyright © 2018 by Shannon Epstein

No part of this publication may be reproduced, stored in a retrieval system or transmitted in any form or by any means, electronic, mechanical, photocopying, recording, scanning or otherwise, except as permitted under Sections 107 or 108 of the 1976 United States Copyright Act, without the prior written permission of the Publisher. Requests to the Publisher for permission should be addressed to the Permissions Department, Rockridge Press, 6005 Shellmound Street, Suite 175, Emeryville, CA 94608.

Limit of Liability/Disclaimer of Warranty: The Publisher and the author make no representations or warranties with respect to the accuracy or completeness of the contents of this work and specifically disclaim all warranties, including without limitation warranties of fitness for a particular purpose. No warranty may be created or extended by sales or promotional materials. The advice and strategies contained herein may not be suitable for every situation. This work is sold with the understanding that the Publisher is not engaged in rendering medical, legal or other professional advice or services. If professional assistance is required, the services of a competent professional person should be sought. Neither the Publisher nor the author shall be liable for damages arising herefrom. The fact that an individual, organization or website is referred to in this work as a citation and/or potential source of further information does not mean that the author or the Publisher endorses the information the individual, organization or website may provide or recommendations they/it may make. Further, readers should be aware that Internet websites listed in this work may have changed or disappeared between when this work was written and when it is read.

For general information on our other products and services or to obtain technical support, please contact our Customer Care Department within the United States at (866) 744-2665, or outside the United States at (510) 253-0500.

Rockridge Press publishes its books in a variety of electronic and print formats. Some content that appears in print may not be available in electronic books, and vice versa.

TRADEMARKS: Rockridge Press and the Rockridge Press logo are trademarks or registered trademarks of Callisto Media Inc. and/or its affiliates, in the United States and other countries, and may not be used without written permission. All other trademarks are the property of their respective owners. Rockridge Press is not associated with any product or vendor mentioned in this book.

Photography © Marija Vidal, 2018

ISBN: Print 978-1-93975-448-6 | eBook 978-1-93975-449-3

Low-Sodium
Slow Cooker Cookbook

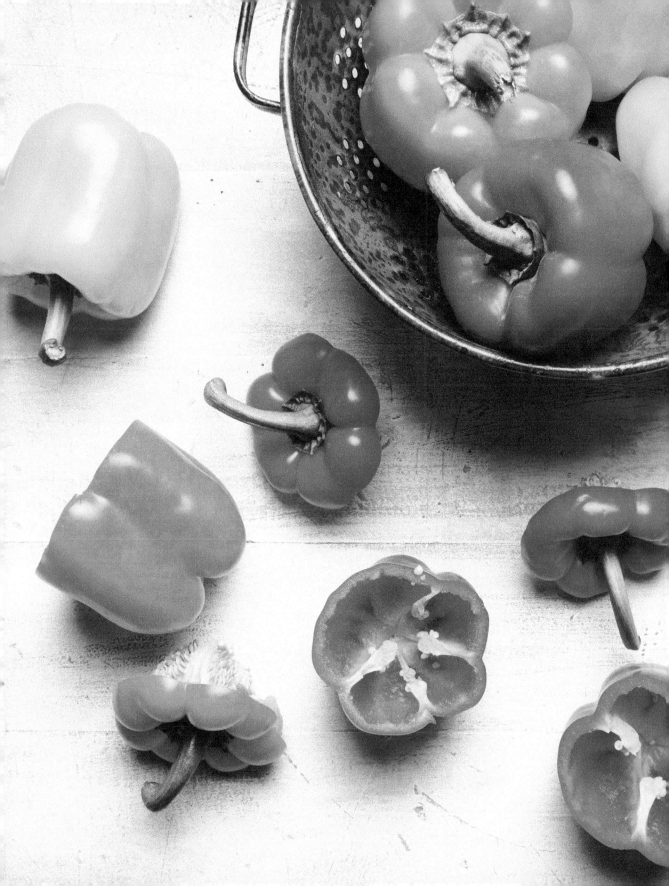

For my parents.
Thank you for your
unconditional
love and support.

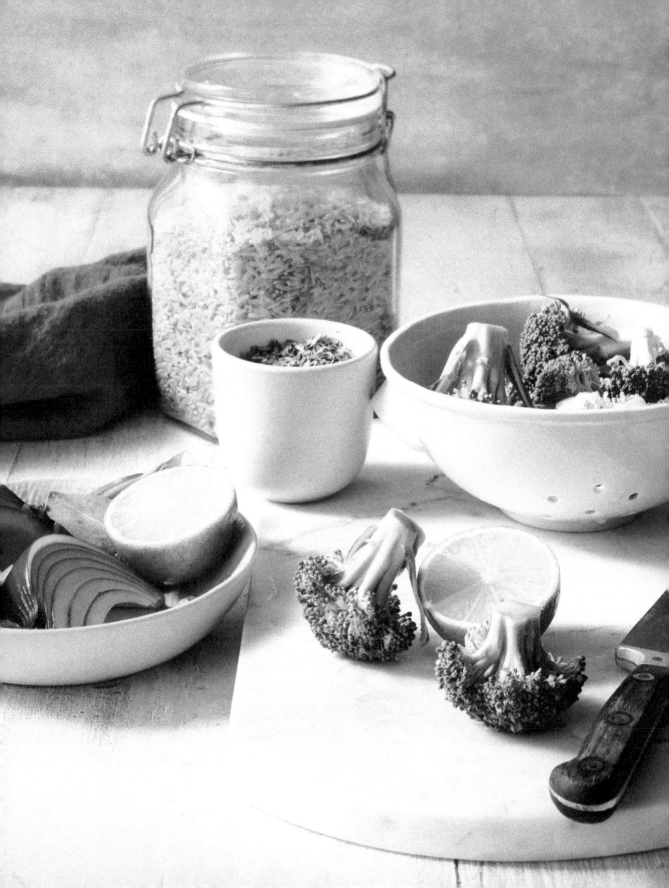

Contents

Introduction

I HOPE YOU'RE READY FOR SOME DELICIOUS RECIPES THAT YOU NEVER would have thought were low-sodium. Whatever your reason for wanting to cut down on salt in your diet—whether it's for you or someone in your family, whether you're addressing a health issue or just trying to eat a bit healthier—you'll find easy recipes here that prep quickly, cook slowly, and are full of flavor.

A little bit about me: I have inadvertently been on a low-sodium diet for years now. I got my first slow cooker as a wedding gift back in 2011. Six months later I found myself at my all-time highest weight . . . with high blood pressure. High blood pressure and heart disease are prevalent on the paternal side of my family. My father has been on high blood pressure medicine for more than 30 years, and my younger brother was hospitalized due to congestive heart failure at the age of 25. When I heard that I, too, had high blood pressure, I knew I needed to make a change. I also knew my future was within my own control.

"Follow a low-sodium diet" was one of the recommendations my brother received when he left the hospital, and it always stuck with me. At the time I was working strict corporate hours, which meant I was eating out at least once a day. And to be honest, when I did cook, it was often some sort of processed food combined with what I thought was something healthy, such as store-bought salad dressing or brown rice that had been preseasoned or covered in a sauce. After a bit of research, though, I realized I needed to start cooking my own meals to be able to control what was in my food.

Then I remembered the slow cooker on the top shelf of my kitchen cabinet. I got it down and started experimenting. Eventually, I started a blog, *Fit Slow Cooker Queen*, to share my unique approach to slow cooking. The majority of the recipes on my blog (including some of the most popular, like my gumbo and steak fajitas) are low-sodium—people just don't realize it. That's because eating low-sodium doesn't mean you have to compromise on flavor; the flavors just come from ingredients other than salt. Cooking this way will improve your health, and without any compromises.

To me, the art of slow cooking is really about minimal prep. Personally, I (generally) don't think it's necessary to take the time to sauté or brown ingredients before you toss them into the slow cooker. I also make every effort to use ingredients that are lean, low-fat, and whole-grain. You can use your slow cooker to create easy, healthy recipes that you'll actually enjoy; I'll show you how.

We're a household of two (these days I cook for my husband and myself almost every day of the week), and obviously I love slow cooking. If you're familiar with the slow cooker, you may be aware that portion control can be a bit tricky to master. Many of the recipes here have four servings, which in my home means they are meant for two meals. That could mean dinner tomorrow or the night after, the next day's lunch, or popping two portions into the freezer. Less work, more flavor!

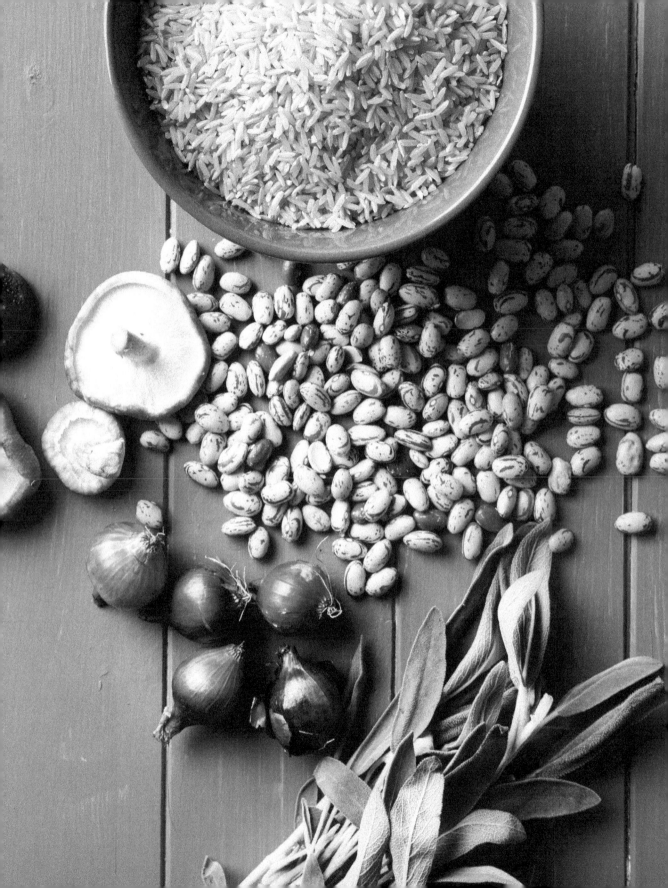

Low-Sodium
SLOW COOKING

The slow cooker is the perfect tool for low-sodium recipes. Cooking food all in one pot using the low and slow method enhances the natural flavors, so a lot of salt is not needed. But this is a cookbook, not a diet book, and I'll be focusing on how to get the most flavor from your ingredients and make meals your family will love. I'll also give you a rundown of essential tools and some shopping guidelines, including how to choose a slow cooker if you don't already have one. And I'll talk about managing a low-sodium diet.

Why Worry About Salt?

We need salt for achieving a normal fluid balance in the body and maintaining normal nerve and muscle functions. But too much salt can be a bad thing. It causes the body to retain too much water. And when that happens, the heart must work harder and blood pressure may increase.

High blood pressure can cause:

- Chest pain
- Damaged/narrowed arteries
- Coronary artery disease
- Kidney failure
- Heart failure
- Stroke

Scary, right? The good news is that in many cases, blood pressure can be controlled with lifestyle changes, including changing your diet to one that's lower in sodium.

BLOOD PRESSURE AND YOU

High blood pressure, also called *hypertension*, is one of the primary reasons people switch to a low-sodium diet. It's caused by too much pressure (tension) in the arteries, the vessels that carry oxygenated blood from the heart to the rest of the body.

When you have your blood pressure taken, it's expressed using two numbers: for example, 120/80. The first number (systolic) is pressure in your arteries when your heart contracts. The second number (diastolic) is the pressure when your heart is between beats.

The American Heart Association recognizes five blood pressure categories. These are for measures that are consistent over several readings:

- Normal: less than 120/80
- Elevated: 129/80
- Hypertension stage 1: 130-139/80-89
- Hypertension stage 2: 140/90 or higher
- Hypertensive crisis: higher than 180/120

Don't Be SAD, Get Healthy

Are you familiar with the Standard American Diet (SAD)? Even if you've never heard of it, statistically speaking, there's a good chance you follow it. In general, the SAD consists of foods that are high in saturated and animal fats, highly processed foods, genetically or chemically altered foods, and foods high in sugar and low in plant foods, fiber, and complex carbohydrates.

Sadly, the SAD diet is one of the main causes of disease in America today. Following this diet can lead to a host of health problems, including:

- Hypertension
- Heart disease
- Stroke
- Obesity
- Diabetes
- Dementia
- Some types of cancer

If you follow the SAD diet, what you are eating is literally making you sick. Again, the good news is that you can immediately improve your overall health by simply changing the way you eat. Including more of the following foods in your diet will positively affect your overall well-being:

- **Fruits** are a good source of many nutrients, including minerals, potassium, fiber, vitamin C, and folic acid.
- **Vegetables** are naturally high-fiber, low-fat, low-calorie, and cholesterol-free. They're also a good source of many nutrients, including potassium, dietary fiber, folic acid, vitamin A, and vitamin C.
- **Legumes** are known for being an excellent source of complex carbohydrates, protein, and fiber, and they also help you feel fuller longer. That means that eating small amounts of legumes can help prevent unwanted or unhealthy snacking.
- **Starchy vegetables**, such as sweet potatoes and winter squash, are a good source of energy. They also contain fiber, calcium, iron, and B vitamins.

- **Whole grains** are an excellent source of fiber and nutrients, including vitamins, minerals, and protein. They also help prevent heart disease and stroke.
- **Lean white meats**, such as chicken and turkey breasts, are a good source of protein, and they have less fat and cholesterol and fewer calories than fattier meats and cuts. Reduce your red meat intake to just a few meals a week, and go for the lean white meats instead.

LABEL SMARTS

The FDA recommends consuming no more than 2,400 mg of sodium per day. The majority of sodium in the SAD comes from processed, premade foods. I understand it's not realistic to think everyone will cook all their own meals, and limiting sodium can be challenging in our SAD world. However, learning to correctly inter-pret nutritional labels will help you choose more wisely and manage your sodium intake.

The Nutrition Facts label on prepared food packages shows the amount of sodium in milligrams (mg) and the Percent Daily Value (%DV) in one serving of the food. When looking at the label, choose foods with a low %DV of sodium. Take a good look at the serving size, because one package of a frozen entrée or what looks like a single-serving bag of chips may actually be labeled as two servings or even more.

Look for products containing less than 100% of the daily value for sodium in a single serving. And in general, look for the low-, light-, or reduced-sodium version of prepared foods. If sodium or salt is listed among the ingredients, definitely avoid that food!

Here's a little secret about blood pressure and diet: Eating more potas-sium causes you to lose more sodium in your urine. Potassium also helps to ease the tension in the walls of your blood vessels. So eating foods that are high in potassium (think bananas, apricots, dates, and beans) can help your blood pressure by reducing the effects of sodium.

Why Slow Cook?

As you can guess, I use my slow cooker a lot. To me, slow cooking is a wonderful, easy way to put wholesome meals on the table. However, I understand that when you think of low-sodium meals, the slow cooker is not the first thing that comes to mind. It's time to rethink that. Slow cookers are a great tool for making healthy meals with minimal fuss. How?

VERSATILITY

Fresh vegetables, a variety of potatoes and winter squash, and pretty much any cut of meat work very well in the slow cooker. Slow cookers let you use less expensive ingredients. For example, using dry beans and just soaking them overnight is not only healthier but cheaper, too.

MINIMAL PREP

Throw the ingredients in and let them cook—that's the slow cooker way! Not only will you save time, but you will have a lot fewer pots and pans to clean up as well. The recipes here are great for when you need to clean out your produce drawer, too—grab your veggies, chop them up, and throw them into the slow cooker.

COOK AND FREEZE

If you want or need to make your meals in advance, most of the recipes in this book are freezer-friendly. If you spend a couple hours prepping freezer meals for the week, you'll be more likely to keep your low-sodium diet on track.

GREAT FLAVOR, BETTER TEXTURE

A slow cooker brings out the flavor in foods—so much flavor, in fact, that you can cook with a lot less salt and sugar. Slow cooking also delivers melt-in-your-mouth meat! The low and slow method of the slow cooker produces meat so tender you can shred it with a fork. The best part is that even the cheapest, toughest cuts of meat will cook up tender and delicious.

MAXIMIZE THE NUTRIENTS

Cooking food at low temperatures for a long time preserves nutrients that are normally lost when food is cooked at high temperatures. Slow cooking also eliminates the risk of AGEs (advanced glycation end products), which form when foods are cooked at high heat and are known to contribute to increased oxidative stress and inflammation, which have been linked to diabetes and cardiovascular disease.

AVOID TEMPTATION

When you throw everything in your slow cooker in the morning and head out for work, you know you're going to come home to a cooked meal (and probably an amazing-smelling house). This will help you avoid eating out or stopping for takeout as often—thus avoiding all the temptations of a restaurant menu.

Slow Cooking Tips and Tricks

While slow cooking is a very easy technique, there are a few tips and tricks you'll need to keep in mind:

- Chop food in large chunks, particularly vegetables and potatoes. This will keep them from falling apart when they get very soft.
- Make sure to cut the meat and vegetables into pieces that are all about the same size, so they cook evenly.

- Cut to fit. If your roast is too big, cut it into two pieces. Do the same for vegetables and even noodles.
- Use frozen vegetables by layering appropriately. Place firm root vegetables (think potatoes) at the bottom of the slow cooker, then the meat, then the frozen vegetables on top.
- Don't remove the lid; set it and forget it. Lifting the lid releases heat—so much that you have to add as much as 30 minutes additional cooking time just from taking a quick peek!
- Don't overcrowd the slow cooker. This will lead to food cooking unevenly or not all the way through.
- Ditch the premade dressing, sauce, and seasoning packets and make your own. You can do this easily, using simple seasonings and spices that you probably already have in your pantry. (You'll find some examples starting on the next page.) Same flavor, way less sodium.
- To brown or not to brown the meat before you add it to the slow cooker? Some people argue that it adds flavor. I'm not 100 percent convinced that's the case, so I usually think of any browning or searing as an optional step.

Flavoring the Low-Sodium Way

At first, sticking to a low-sodium diet can make seasoning difficult. You're not adding salt, and many store-bought products, like seasoning packets and dressings, are high in sodium. The answer is to make them yourself. I think you'll find that their homemade replacements are just as good, if not better.

Herbs, whether fresh or dried, and more unusual spices like curry or basic seasonings like cumin, can do wonders for a dish. The combination possibilities are endless, and you can tailor the flavors to your tastes. Like spicy? Make chili powder your base for a nice, spicy blend. Homemade blends add so much flavor, all without any added sodium.

Below I've included a few spice blends and salad dressings to get you started. I keep a jar of each of the blends in my pantry and a bottle of dressing in my fridge, so I have them ready to use all the time.

HOMEMADE FAJITA BLEND

1 tablespoon chili powder

1½ teaspoons ground cumin

1 teaspoon freshly ground
 black pepper

1 teaspoon salt

½ teaspoon paprika

½ teaspoon dried oregano

¼ teaspoon garlic powder

¼ teaspoon onion powder

¼ teaspoon red pepper flakes

In a jar, combine the chili powder, cumin, pepper, salt, paprika, oregano, garlic powder, onion powder, and red pepper flakes. Put the lid on, and shake it up.

HOMEMADE CAJUN BLEND

4 teaspoons salt

4 teaspoons garlic powder

3 teaspoons dried oregano

2 teaspoons freshly ground
 black pepper

2 teaspoons onion powder

2 teaspoons ground cayenne pepper

2 teaspoons dried thyme

2 teaspoons red pepper flakes

In a jar, combine the salt, garlic powder, oregano, pepper, onion powder, cayenne, thyme, and red pepper flakes. Put the lid on, and shake it up.

HOMEMADE ITALIAN BLEND

2 tablespoons dried basil

2 tablespoons dried oregano

2 tablespoons dried parsley

2 tablespoons ground coriander

2 tablespoons dried thyme

2 teaspoons freshly ground
   black pepper

2 teaspoons garlic powder

2 teaspoons onion powder

2 teaspoons red pepper flakes

In a jar, combine the basil, oregano, parsley, coriander, thyme, pepper, garlic powder, onion powder, and red pepper flakes. Put the lid on, and shake it up.

HOMEMADE DRY RANCH DRESSING MIX

2 tablespoons dried chopped onions

1 tablespoon dried parsley

1 tablespoon dried chives

1 tablespoon dried dill

2 teaspoons garlic powder

2 teaspoons onion powder

1 teaspoon salt

In a jar, combine the onions, parsley, chives, dill, garlic powder, onion powder, and salt. Put the lid on, and shake it up.

HOMEMADE DRY ONION SOUP MIX

¼ cup dried chopped onions

2 tablespoons onion powder

1 tablespoon dried parsley

1 teaspoon ground turmeric

1 teaspoon salt

1 teaspoon garlic powder

½ teaspoon freshly ground
   black pepper

In a jar, combine the onions, onion powder, parsley, turmeric, salt, garlic powder, and pepper. Put the lid on, and shake it up.

HOMEMADE ITALIAN VINAIGRETTE

½ cup extra-virgin olive oil

¼ cup red wine vinegar

1 teaspoon dried oregano

½ teaspoon salt

½ teaspoon freshly ground
 black pepper

¼ teaspoon garlic powder

In a large bowl, whisk to combine the olive oil, vinegar, oregano, salt, pepper, and garlic powder until well blended. Store in a bottle or jar in the refrigerator.

CILANTRO-LIME DRESSING

1 bunch fresh cilantro, stemmed

½ cup plain fat-free Greek yogurt

2 garlic cloves, minced

2 tablespoons apple cider vinegar

2 tablespoons extra-virgin olive oil

Juice of 1 lime (2 to 3 tablespoons)

Pinch salt

In a blender or food processor, blend to combine the cilantro, yogurt, garlic, vinegar, olive oil, lime juice, and salt until smooth. Store in a bottle or jar in the refrigerator.

Equipment Basics

You don't need a lot of equipment for slow cooker cuisine, but there are some basics. I'll bet you already have most of these items on hand.

A FAITHFUL APPLIANCE

Of course, you must have a slow cooker. In general, slow cookers come in under 2 quarts, 3.5 quarts, 4, 5, or 6 quarts, and 7 quarts or larger. For the recipes in this cookbook, you'll never need more than a 3.5-quart slow cooker.

It can be tricky to use a slow cooker that's too big for the amount of food you're cooking. If you don't have enough food to fill the slow cooker at least three-quarters full, you risk burning your meal.

If you already have a larger slow cooker (or a larger family!), you may not need to buy a smaller one; you could just cook more food. Most of the recipes in this cookbook can easily be doubled or even tripled to serve more.

Personally, even though we're a household of two, I cook for four every day so my husband and I have leftovers for lunch. It's healthier than take-out, and it's cheaper, too. And if you want to fill your freezer with stacks of single-serving home-cooked meals, a bigger cooker may be right for you.

Another way to correct for size is by using slow cooker liners or bags. As long as you fill the bag, you don't have to worry about the entire cooker being full. You can find slow cooker liners at your local grocery store or online.

OTHER NECESSARY EQUIPMENT

Immersion blender or blender. You'll need this to blend soups and some other dishes. Personally, I like to use an immersion blender because you don't have to transfer the liquid to a blender; you blend it directly in the slow cooker.

Nonstick cooking spray and parchment paper. Lots of ingredients, like eggs, rice, cheese, and batter, tend to stick to the slow cooker while cooking. You'll need these to ensure that doesn't happen.

Knives and knife sharpener. A couple of simple straight-edge knives are all you need for any recipe in this cookbook. Get a longer, heavier one and a shorter one. Those knives must be sharp, so grab a knife sharpener, too. The handheld kind with a guide that you pull your knife through is very easy to use and inexpensive.

Cutting boards. Slow cooking involves chopping, so you'll need a surface for that. Get a minimum of two—one for vegetables and one for meats. If you can, get an additional cutting board so you can separate poultry from red meat. Plastic ones in different colors will help you remember which board is for which food. Please wash them thoroughly after each use, especially after handling raw meat.

Plan It Out

The best way to stick to a low-sodium diet is to plan out your meals for the week. When you're prepared, you're less likely to slip up.

Keeping your sodium intake limit in mind, decide what you'll have for each meal of the day, including any snacks. Planning your meals will not only make you more aware of the nutritional values of the food you're eating, but it will also help you stay on track. If you have a set menu, you're less likely to end up ordering takeout.

There are tons of free online tools and apps out there that you can use to track your meal plans, along with nutritional values of individual foods. Some of the ones I like are MyFitnessPal, FitDaily, and MyFoodDiary. With a little bit of research, I'm sure you'll be able to find one that fits your needs.

Here are some other simple meal planning strategies:

- Create a weekly menu. Write out what you're going to eat for each meal. Use it to compile your grocery list, and buy only the ingredients on the list.
- Make recipes that you can eat over a couple days. Casseroles and slow cooker meals are especially good for this.
- Cook in bulk. Roast a couple pounds of chicken at once and use it throughout the rest of the week in salads, sandwiches, or casseroles.
- Double your recipes, and eat the leftovers for lunch the next day.
- Freeze slow cooker meals in smaller servings for up to six months.

SAMPLE MEAL PLAN

Below, you'll find a week-long meal plan that incorporates the recipes in this book. You'll notice many of the lunch meals are leftovers from dinner the night before. If you have strict limitations on your daily sodium intake, pay close attention to the sodium values given in the nutrition info at the end of each recipe and plan accordingly. Because many of these recipes have a long cook time, due to the nature of slow cooking, I recommend making your breakfast meals the night before, and enjoying leftovers as necessary!

MONDAY

Breakfast - Protein Oatmeal Bake (page 41)

Lunch - Gazpacho (page 76)

Dinner - Zucchini Casserole (page 96)

Dessert - Sweet Granola Clusters (page 155)

TUESDAY

Breakfast - Breakfast Scramble (page 46)

Lunch - Leftover Zucchini Casserole

Dinner -Herbed Pork Loin (page 142)

Dessert - Leftover Sweet Granola Clusters

WEDNESDAY

Breakfast - Cheese Grits (page 42)

Lunch - Stuffed Acorn Squash (page 105)

Dinner - Chicken Tortilla Soup (page 84)

Dessert - Leftover Sweet Granola Clusters

THURSDAY

Breakfast - Eggs with Green Bell
   Peppers and Diced Tomatoes
   (page 45)

Lunch - Leftover Chicken
   Tortilla Soup

Dinner - Beef Goulash (page 147)

Dessert - Zucchini Brownies
   (page 157)

FRIDAY

Breakfast - Oatmeal (page 40)

Lunch - Leftover Beef Goulash

Dinner - Enchilada Quinoa Bake
   (page 67)

Dessert - Leftover Zucchini Brownies

SATURDAY

Breakfast - Egg White Vegetable
   Frittata (page 44)

Lunch - Gumbo (page 90)

Dinner - Filipino Pork Adobo
   (page 143)

Dessert - Blueberry Cobbler
   (page 160)

SUNDAY

Breakfast - French Toast (page 43)

Lunch - Green Curry Vegetable
   Soup (page 80)

Dinner - Leftover Filipino Pork Adobo

Dessert - Leftover Blueberry Cobbler

Healthy Ingredients for a Healthier You

Although canned or prepackaged food can make prepping and cooking simpler, I recommend using seasonal, fresh, and organic produce. To start, these ingredients contain fewer pesticides. Chemicals that are used in agriculture can remain on food even after a good washing. Organic produce is usually also fresher because it is grown locally.

It's the same for meat and poultry. Try to find organically produced fresh meats, from animals that are not given antibiotics or hormones. Organic food is generally GMO-free. Avoid cured meats like bacon and salami, as they are usually high in sodium.

Frozen produce is okay, too. Most frozen fruits and veggies are blanched and frozen within hours of being picked. This helps lock in freshness and nutritional value. Frozen produce is also available year-round and is usually cheaper than fresh. Look for frozen produce with no added sauces or flavors of any kind—and, of course, no added salt.

Here are four "great for slow cooking" foods, one for each season:

Spring: Apples are fragrant, sweet, and delicious, and they can be used in everything from beverages to main dishes to desserts.

Summer: Tomatoes can make or break a slow cooker recipe. They can be used as a base, a sauce, a main ingredient, or flavor enhancement. While fresh tomatoes are at their peak in the summer, good no-salt-added canned ones are available year-round.

Fall: Potatoes are one of my favorite ingredients to slow cook. They hold up very well over the long cooking time, and they provide a basic yet nutritional starch element to a dish.

Winter: Cabbage is a sturdy vegetable, so it withstands long cooking as well. It also takes in seasonings very well, so when slow cooked with the right spices it can be a very flavorful ingredient.

PRODUCE STORAGE TIPS

Follow these simple tips to help your produce last longer in the refrigerator, so you won't end up buying things and then throwing them out:

- To combat mold, don't wash your berries until you're ready to use them.
- Store unripe fruits and vegetables out on the counter at room temperature. To slow down ripening, move the produce to the refrigerator.
- Store citrus in a cool, dark place, away from direct sunlight. To slow down ripening, move it to the refrigerator.
- Store potatoes, onions, and tomatoes in a cool, dry place at room temperature.
- Store lettuce in a separate bag in the produce drawer with a paper towel tucked around it. Eat it soon, because it tends to spoil very quickly.

About the Recipes

For the most part, I want to let the ingredients in these recipes speak for themselves. I used the lowest-sodium ingredients that made each dish work, and you'll notice there's very little added salt in each recipe—sometimes none at all.

For your ease in planning, each recipe follows what I call a sodium scale, tagged either low (251+ milligrams of sodium), lower (101 to 250 milligrams), or lowest (0 to 100 milligrams). Many of the staple recipes in chapter 2, like bone broth, vegetable broth, and chicken broth, will fall into the lowest sodium category, while recipes that include a sauce, like the Enchilada Quinoa Bake (page 67), will be categorized as low.

It's important for me (and you!) to keep prep to a minimum with every recipe. You won't find a recipe that involves more than 15 minutes of prep, and that's leaving plenty of time for everything.

From low-sodium stews and soups to vegetarian and vegan recipes, roasts, and casseroles, there is something for everyone here. Overall, I think you'll be pleasantly surprised with the amount of flavor the dishes have.

RECIPE LABELS

We all have our own tastes and dietary needs. That's why each recipe has the following labels, so you can make sure whichever one you choose will best meet your needs. Of course, for these recipe labels to be accurate, you'll need to make sure the brand of any store-bought products you use complies with your dietary restrictions. For example, a recipe containing Worcestershire sauce and labeled Vegan, Gluten-Free, and Allergy-Friendly will only be vegan if the sauce you use contains no anchovies, gluten-free if the sauce is gluten-free, and allergy-friendly if the sauce is free of anchovies, wheat, and soy protein.

Allergy-Friendly: The recipe does not contain any of the "big 8" allergens, which account for 90 percent of food allergic reactions: dairy, eggs, fish, crustaceans, tree nuts, peanuts, wheat, and soybeans.

Gluten-Free: The recipe does not include any gluten.

Low-Carb: The recipe contains only 30 grams of carbohydrates or less per serving.

Low-Cholesterol: The recipe contains only 20 milligrams of cholesterol or less per serving.

Vegan: The recipe does not contain any products derived from animals.

Vegetarian: The recipe does not include any meat, but does have dairy and/or eggs.

All recipes are low-sodium, low-fat, and heart-healthy, and they all include full nutrition information so you can make the best decisions for your health.

Give Yourself Some Time

Any type of change can be hard. If you're adapting to a low-sodium lifestyle for the first time, it can definitely be difficult. You may miss the sodium at first. Don't give up! Over time, you won't miss it as much. Just remember, change doesn't happen overnight.

Think of your journey as slow and steady. The best thing to do is take it one meal at a time. If you fall off track, all you have to do is get back on at the next meal. Even replacing one meal with a low-sodium option is better than nothing at all. You'll see improvement in your health, which will make the effort worth it. I promise!

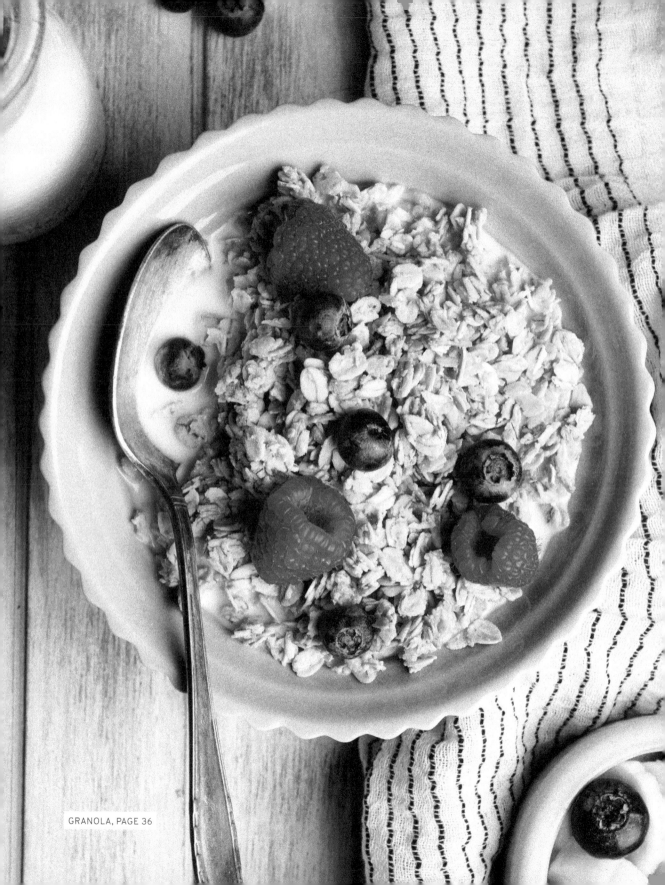

GRANOLA, PAGE 36

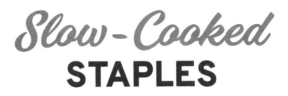

Slow-Cooked STAPLES

Vegetable Broth

MAKES 8 CUPS • **PREP TIME:** 10 MINUTES • **COOK TIME:** 8 TO 10 HOURS ON LOW

LOWEST SODIUM

ALLERGY-FRIENDLY • GLUTEN-FREE • LOW-CARB • LOW-CHOLESTEROL • VEGAN

Vegetable broth can be used in so many recipes, including any recipe in this book that calls for broth. Whether as a base of a soup or in a gravy, it's so versatile. Because this broth is meat-free, it can be used in pretty much any recipe regardless of your diet. There is no added salt; all the flavor comes from the vegetables, herbs, and spices.

8 cups water

3 large onions, chopped

5 garlic cloves, minced

5 carrots, chopped

4 celery stalks, chopped

¼ cup chopped fresh parsley

4 thyme or rosemary sprigs

3 dried bay leaves

½ teaspoon whole peppercorns

1. In the slow cooker, combine the water, onions, garlic, carrots, celery, parsley, thyme, bay leaves, and peppercorns.
2. Cook on low for 8 to 10 hours.
3. Strain the solids from the broth using a large mesh strainer. Using the back of a spoon, press the excess liquid from the vegetables in the strainer.

STORAGE TIP: This broth (and the others in this chapter) can be stored in the refrigerator for 3 to 5 days or frozen for up to 6 months.

PER SERVING (1 CUP) Calories: 16; Total Fat: 0g; Saturated Fat: 0g; Cholesterol: 0mg; Sodium: 87mg; Potassium: 0mg; Carbs: 2g; Fiber: 0g; Protein: 0g

Chicken Broth

MAKES 8 CUPS • **PREP TIME:** 10 MINUTES • **COOK TIME:** 8 TO 10 HOURS ON LOW

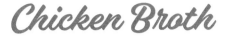 LOWEST SODIUM

ALLERGY-FRIENDLY • GLUTEN-FREE • LOW-CARB • LOW-CHOLESTEROL

Slow cooking your leftover bones from a roasted chicken, along with vegetables, water, herbs, and spices, extracts their gelatin and flavor, which produces a savory, rich homemade broth. Just a pinch of salt and pepper is all you need. The rest of the flavor comes from the bones and vegetables. You can store chicken carcasses in the freezer until you have enough for soup. You can use this broth in any recipe in the book that calls for chicken broth.

3 to 5 pounds leftover chicken carcass bones

8 cups water

5 celery stalks, chopped

5 carrots, chopped

5 garlic cloves, minced

2 large onions, chopped

¼ cup chopped fresh parsley

Pinch salt

Pinch freshly ground black pepper

1. In the slow cooker, combine the bones, water, celery, carrots, garlic, onions, parsley, salt, and pepper.
2. Cook on low for 8 to 10 hours.
3. Strain the solids from the broth using a large mesh strainer.

VARIATION: Use whatever fresh herbs you have. Feel free to add other vegetables as well. The important thing is to keep the base of chicken bones, carrots, and onions.

PER SERVING (1 CUP) Calories: 38; Total Fat: 1g; Saturated Fat: 0g; Cholesterol: 0mg; Sodium: 52mg; Potassium: 131mg; Carbs: 3g; Fiber: 0g; Protein: 5g

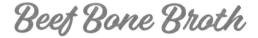

Beef Bone Broth

MAKES 8 CUPS • **PREP TIME:** 5 MINUTES • **COOK TIME:** 20 TO 24 HOURS ON LOW

LOWER SODIUM

ALLERGY-FRIENDLY • GLUTEN-FREE • LOW-CARB • LOW-CHOLESTEROL

Bone broth has tons of nutritional value, but it does take time to extract all those nutrients. Homemade bone broth needs to cook for a long time, which makes it the perfect slow cooker recipe. The measurements don't have to be exact. In fact, my best batches come out when I'm just throwing the ingredients in there. You can use this broth in any recipe in the book that calls for beef broth.

4 pounds beef bones (such as oxtail, short ribs, or neck bones)

8 cups water

4 celery stalks, chopped

4 carrots, chopped

2 onions, chopped

5 garlic cloves, minced

¼ cup white vinegar

½ teaspoon salt

½ teaspoon freshly ground black pepper

1 dried bay leaf

1. In the slow cooker, combine the bones, water, celery, carrots, onions, garlic, vinegar, salt, pepper, and bay leaf.
2. Cook on low for 20 to 24 hours.
3. Strain the solids from the broth using a large mesh strainer.

INGREDIENT TIP: If the bones are fatty, place your broth in the refrigerator overnight. In the morning, remove the layer of fat that has solidified on the top.

PER SERVING (1 CUP) Calories: 22; Total Fat: 0g; Saturated Fat: 0g; Cholesterol: 0mg; Sodium: 167mg; Potassium: 54mg; Carbs: 1g; Fiber: 0g; Protein: 2g

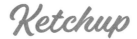

Ketchup

MAKES 4 CUPS • **PREP TIME:** 5 MINUTES • **COOK TIME:** 4 TO 6 HOURS ON LOW

LOWER SODIUM

ALLERGY-FRIENDLY • GLUTEN-FREE • LOW-CARB • LOW-CHOLESTEROL • VEGETARIAN

My family's roots are in Pittsburgh, so I take my ketchup very seriously. Even though I removed all the added sugar, I think you'll find this healthier version is just as good as the store-bought variety. It'll keep for about 3 weeks in the refrigerator or 6 months in the freezer.

5 pounds Roma tomatoes (fresh or no-salt-added canned), sliced

1 small onion, diced

2 garlic cloves, minced

¼ cup honey

¼ cup apple cider vinegar

1 tablespoon ground mustard

1 teaspoon salt

½ teaspoon gluten-free Worcestershire sauce

¼ teaspoon freshly ground black pepper

¼ teaspoon ground cinnamon

¼ teaspoon paprika

1. In the slow cooker, combine the tomatoes, onion, garlic, honey, vinegar, ground mustard, salt, Worcestershire sauce, pepper, cinnamon, and paprika. Stir to mix well.

2. Cook on low for 4 to 6 hours.

3. Carefully transfer the sauce to a blender or use an immersion blender to purée to your desired consistency.

VARIATION: If you like your ketchup on the sweeter side, add a tad more honey.

PER SERVING (¼ CUP) Calories: 48; Total Fat: 0g; Saturated Fat: 0g; Cholesterol: 0mg; Sodium: 154mg; Potassium: 356mg; Carbs: 11g; Fiber: 2g; Protein: 2g

Gravy

MAKES 4 CUPS • **PREP TIME:** 5 MINUTES • **COOK TIME:** 4 HOURS 15 MINUTES
TO 6 HOURS 15 MINUTES ON LOW

LOWEST SODIUM

GLUTEN-FREE • LOW-CARB • LOW-CHOLESTEROL • VEGETARIAN

The fact that this gravy is homemade and not from a can is already a good start. This version does not contain meat drippings, so it can be used in vegetarian recipes as well. It also uses ghee, which is clarified butter—the milk fat has been separated and removed. Ghee is more nutrient-dense than butter, and it's also lactose-free. More and more supermarkets are carrying it in the dairy case, right next to the butter.

4 cups any gluten-free
low-sodium broth

2 tablespoons ghee
(clarified butter)

1 small onion, diced

¼ cup low-fat milk

Salt

Freshly ground black pepper

¼ cup cornstarch

½ cup water

1. In the slow cooker, combine the broth, ghee, onion, and milk. Season lightly with salt and pepper, and stir to mix well.

2. Cook on low for 4 to 6 hours.

3. In a large measuring cup, mix together the cornstarch and water. Slowly stir the cornstarch slurry into the slow cooker. Cook on low for an additional 15 minutes, or until the gravy has thickened.

SUBSTITUTION TIP: Substitute almond milk or soy milk for dairy milk, and you'll have a lactose-free gravy. You can also replace the cornstarch with another thickening agent, such as arrowroot flour or potato starch.

PER SERVING (⅛ CUP) Calories: 40; Total Fat: 2g; Saturated Fat: 0g; Cholesterol: 0mg; Sodium: 55mg; Potassium: 18mg; Carbs: 4g; Fiber: 0g; Protein: 0g

Barbecue Sauce

MAKES 8 CUPS • **PREP TIME:** 5 MINUTES • **COOK TIME:** 4 TO 6 HOURS

LOW SODIUM

ALLERGY-FRIENDLY • GLUTEN-FREE • LOW-CARB • LOW-CHOLESTEROL • VEGETARIAN

Barbecue sauce is one of the top condiments in America for a reason. This versatile sauce can be used in all sorts of dishes, whether or not they are actually barbecued. Store-bought barbecue sauces can contain large amounts of both sodium and sugar. Neither is necessary to make a great-tasting sauce, especially when the slow cooker is involved.

4 cups Ketchup (page 25)

2 cups water

¾ cup apple cider vinegar

½ cup maple syrup

2 tablespoons gluten-free Worcestershire sauce

2 tablespoons freshly squeezed lemon juice

2 teaspoons ground mustard

1½ teaspoons salt

1 teaspoon freshly ground black pepper

1 teaspoon onion powder

1. In the slow cooker, combine the ketchup, water, vinegar, syrup, Worcestershire sauce, lemon juice, mustard, salt, pepper, and onion powder. Stir to mix well.

2. Cook on low for 4 to 6 hours.

3. Carefully transfer the sauce to a blender or use an immersion blender to purée to your desired consistency.

VARIATION: Stir in ½ teaspoon of liquid smoke to give this barbecue sauce a smoky flavor.

PER SERVING (½ CUP) Calories: 82; Total Fat: 0g; Saturated Fat: 0g; Cholesterol: 0mg; Sodium: 395mg; Potassium: 416mg; Carbs: 19g; Fiber: 0g; Protein: 2g

Enchilada Sauce

MAKES 4 CUPS • **PREP TIME:** 15 MINUTES • **COOK TIME:** 4 TO 6 HOURS ON LOW, PLUS 15 MINUTES ON HIGH

LOWER SODIUM

ALLERGY-FRIENDLY • LOW-CARB • LOW-CHOLESTEROL • VEGAN

Using simple ingredients, this homemade enchilada sauce can be used on everything from enchiladas to tacos or even in a casserole. This recipe produces a fairly mild enchilada sauce. You can add more chili powder or even ground cayenne pepper if you're looking for something a little spicier. I suggest you taste first before making any additions.

3 tablespoons extra-virgin olive oil

3 tablespoons flour (whole-wheat flour, all-purpose flour, or gluten-free flour blends all work!)

2 cups low-sodium vegetable broth

2 tablespoons chili powder

2 tablespoons no-salt-added tomato paste

1 teaspoon apple cider vinegar or distilled white vinegar

1 teaspoon ground cumin

½ teaspoon garlic powder

¼ teaspoon dried oregano

Salt

Freshly ground black pepper

1. Preheat the slow cooker to high. When it's hot, add the oil and flour. Cook for 15 minutes, stirring frequently until the flour has dissolved.
2. Add the broth, chili powder, tomato paste, vinegar, cumin, garlic powder, and oregano, and season lightly with salt and pepper. Stir to mix well.
3. Cook on low for 4 to 6 hours.
4. Carefully transfer the sauce to a blender or use an immersion blender to purée to your desired consistency.

COOKING TIP: To save time, you can cook the oil and flour on the stove top first and add it to the slow cooker about 15 minutes after the remaining ingredients have already begun cooking.

PER SERVING (½ CUP) Calories: 73; Total Fat: 6g; Saturated Fat: 1g; Cholesterol: 0mg; Sodium: 117mg; Potassium: 96mg; Carbs: 6g; Fiber: 2g; Protein: 1g

Salsa

MAKES 4 CUPS • PREP TIME: 5 MINUTES • COOK TIME: 2 TO 4 HOURS ON LOW

LOWEST SODIUM

ALLERGY-FRIENDLY • GLUTEN-FREE • LOW-CARB • LOW-CHOLESTEROL • VEGAN

This salsa recipe is so easy and good that you might never buy store-bought again. Using fresh ingredients, you'll have restaurant-style salsa made right in your slow cooker. Spice this up by adding some heat, like a diced jalapeño. You can double or triple this recipe for your next party. Your salsa will last in the refrigerator for up to a month.

3 large tomatoes, chopped

1 small onion, chopped

1 bell pepper, seeded and chopped

1 garlic clove, minced

1 tablespoon white vinegar

½ teaspoon salt

½ teaspoon ground cumin

¼ teaspoon freshly ground black pepper

¼ cup chopped fresh cilantro

1. In the slow cooker, combine the tomatoes, onion, bell pepper, garlic, vinegar, salt, cumin, and pepper. Stir to mix well.
2. Cook on low for 2 to 4 hours.
3. Stir in the cilantro, and cool before serving.

VARIATION: For extra flavor, you can drizzle the tomatoes with extra-virgin olive oil and roast in a 400°F oven for about 30 minutes, or until tender, before adding them to the slow cooker. Feel like salsa verde? Use green tomatillos instead of tomatoes.

PER SERVING (½ CUP) Calories: 22; Total Fat: 0g; Saturated Fat: 0g; Cholesterol: 0mg; Sodium: 5mg; Potassium: 214mg; Carbs: 5g; Fiber: 1g; Protein: 1g

Marinara Sauce

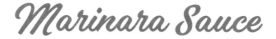

MAKES 4 CUPS • **PREP TIME:** 5 MINUTES • **COOK TIME:** 4 TO 6 HOURS ON LOW

`LOWEST SODIUM`

ALLERGY-FRIENDLY • GLUTEN-FREE • LOW-CARB • LOW-CHOLESTEROL • VEGAN

If you're not careful, buying a store-bought marinara sauce can leave you with a high-sodium, sugar-filled dish of pasta. Making your own marinara sauce is not only super easy, but the combo of tomatoes and fresh herbs simmering on low for hours will make your kitchen smell amazing. You can easily double or triple this recipe, and it's another great one for freezing. If you are going to freeze your sauce, allow it to cool completely first.

3½ pounds Roma
   tomatoes, chopped

4 garlic cloves, minced

¼ cup chopped fresh basil

1½ teaspoons dried oregano

½ teaspoon dried thyme

Salt

Freshly ground black pepper

1. In the slow cooker, combine the tomatoes, garlic, basil, oregano, and thyme, and season lightly with salt and pepper. Stir to mix well.

2. Cook on low for 4 to 6 hours, or until the consistency is to your liking.

3. Carefully transfer the sauce to a blender or use an immersion blender to purée to your desired consistency.

INGREDIENT TIP: Canned whole peeled tomatoes are fine to use here, but try to find a brand that is sugar-free and low-sodium or salt-free.

PER SERVING (1 CUP) Calories: 78; Total Fat: 1g; Saturated Fat: 0g; Cholesterol: 0mg; Sodium: 45mg; Potassium: 970mg; Carbs: 17g; Fiber: 5g; Protein: 4g

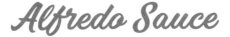

Alfredo Sauce

MAKES 4 CUPS • **PREP TIME:** 5 MINUTES • **COOK TIME:** 4 TO 6 HOURS ON LOW

LOW SODIUM

LOW-CARB • VEGETARIAN

Alfredo sauce can be packed with sodium if you're not careful. This recipe is a prime example of how reducing the sodium doesn't mean you have to strip out the flavor. The elements that make Alfredo sauce are still here, but with half the calories and less than half the salt. If you find that your sauce isn't as thick as you would like, try stirring an additional 1 tablespoon of cornstarch into the slow cooker after the cook time is completed.

3 cups low-fat milk

2 garlic cloves, minced

2 tablespoons cornstarch

¼ cup fat-free cream cheese

¾ cup grated low-fat
Parmesan cheese

1 tablespoon extra-virgin olive oil

Freshly ground black pepper

1. In the slow cooker, combine the milk, garlic, cornstarch, cream cheese, Parmesan cheese, and olive oil, and season with pepper. Stir to mix well.

2. Cook on low for 4 to 6 hours.

3. Carefully transfer the sauce to a blender or use an immersion blender to purée to your desired consistency.

VARIATION: Add a dash of fresh herbs—whatever you like—for a bit of extra flavor.

PER SERVING (1 CUP) Calories: 290; Total Fat: 16g; Saturated Fat: 8g; Cholesterol: 40mg; Sodium: 497mg; Potassium: 390mg; Carbs: 15g; Fiber: 0g; Protein: 16g

Coconut-Curry Sauce

MAKES 4 CUPS • **PREP TIME:** 5 MINUTES • **COOK TIME:** 4 TO 6 HOURS ON LOW

LOWEST SODIUM

GLUTEN-FREE • LOW-CARB • LOW-CHOLESTEROL • VEGETARIAN

This coconut-curry sauce can be used as a base for lots of recipes—curries or not. You can add this sauce to a salad dressing, use it as a base for a soup, or use it as a condiment for dipping. For a lighter version, substitute light coconut milk. To mix things up, you can add fresh herbs, too: ¼ cup of fresh basil makes a nice variation.

2 (15-ounce) cans full-fat coconut milk

3 tablespoons curry paste

1 tablespoon low-sodium soy sauce (or tamari if gluten-free)

4 garlic cloves, coarsely chopped

2 teaspoons honey (optional, omit if vegan)

1½ teaspoons ground ginger

1. In the slow cooker, combine the coconut milk, curry paste, soy sauce, garlic, honey (if using), and ginger. Stir to mix well.

2. Cook on low for 4 to 6 hours.

3. Carefully transfer the sauce to a blender or use an immersion blender to purée to your desired consistency.

STORAGE TIP: Store this sauce in the refrigerator for up to 3 days, or you can freeze it for up to 6 months.

PER SERVING (½ CUP) Calories: 216; Total Fat: 23g; Saturated Fat: 20g; Cholesterol: 0mg; Sodium: 81mg; Potassium: 261mg; Carbs: 5g; Fiber: 1g; Protein: 3g

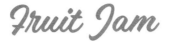

Fruit Jam

MAKES 2 CUPS • **PREP TIME:** 5 MINUTES • **COOK TIME:** 2 TO 4 HOURS ON LOW

LOWEST SODIUM

ALLERGY-FRIENDLY • GLUTEN-FREE • LOW-CARB • LOW-CHOLESTEROL • VEGETARIAN

I'm purposely leaving the name of this recipe vague, because you can use so many different types of fruit for it: apples, blueberries, strawberries, apricots, or anything else you like. Whatever jam you normally buy in the store, you can most likely make a healthier version at home in the slow cooker. Use the natural sweetener that fits your dietary lifestyle. For example, if you're vegan, use natural maple syrup rather than honey.

1 pound fruit, sliced (skin-on)

2 tablespoons water

2 tablespoons honey (or maple syrup if vegan)

1. In the slow cooker, combine the fruit, water, and honey. Stir to mix well.

2. Cook on low for 2 to 4 hours.

3. Carefully transfer the jam to a blender or use an immersion blender to purée to your desired consistency.

4. Spoon the jam into a container with a lid (a Mason jar is best), cool, and store in the refrigerator.

STORAGE TIP: Jam can be stored in an air-tight container in the refrigerator for up to 2 weeks.

PER SERVING (⅛ CUP) Calories: 45; Total Fat: 0g; Saturated Fat: 0g; Cholesterol: 0mg; Sodium: 1mg; Potassium: 119mg; Carbs: 12g; Fiber: 2g; Protein: 1g

Applesauce

MAKES 6 CUPS • **PREP TIME:** 5 MINUTES • **COOK TIME:** 4 TO 6 HOURS ON LOW

LOWEST SODIUM

ALLERGY-FRIENDLY • GLUTEN-FREE • LOW-CARB • LOW-CHOLESTEROL • VEGAN

A lot of slow cooker applesauce recipes use sugar, but it's absolutely not needed. Using the right apples provides enough natural sweetness. For example, Gala and Red Delicious are great choices for this recipe because they're both on the sweeter side. Leave the skin on! The slow cooker will reduce every part of the apple to softness, including the skin.

3 pounds apples, cored and sliced

¼ cup water

2 teaspoons ground cinnamon

1. In the slow cooker, combine the apples, water, and cinnamon. Stir to mix well.
2. Cook on low for 4 to 6 hours.
3. Carefully transfer the sauce to a blender or use an immersion blender to purée to your desired consistency.

VARIATION: To sweeten this sauce without using any added sugar, try adding a teaspoon or two of honey or natural maple syrup. You can even add three or four chopped dates.

PER SERVING (¾ CUP) Calories: 90; Total Fat: 0g; Saturated Fat: 0g; Cholesterol: 0mg; Sodium: 2mg; Potassium: 185mg; Carbs: 24g; Fiber: 4g; Protein: 0g

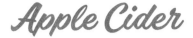

Apple Cider

MAKES 8 CUPS • **PREP TIME:** 15 MINUTES • **COOK TIME:** 4 TO 6 HOURS ON LOW

LOWEST SODIUM

ALLERGY-FRIENDLY • GLUTEN-FREE • LOW-CARB • LOW-CHOLESTEROL • VEGETARIAN

Homemade cider is one of those slow cooker recipes that will have your kitchen smelling amazing after just a few hours. It's also one of those recipes that prove that with the right ingredients, you can ditch the added sugar.

3 pounds apples, cored and sliced

¼ cup honey (or maple syrup if vegan)

½ teaspoon ground nutmeg

3 to 4 cinnamon sticks or ½ teaspoon ground cinnamon

1. In the slow cooker, combine the apples, honey, nutmeg, and cinnamon. Add enough water to cover the apples.
2. Cook on low for 4 to 6 hours, or until the apples are soft.
3. Directly in the slow cooker, mash the softened apples with a potato masher or a wooden spoon.
4. Set a medium pot in the sink. Over the pot, strain the mashed fruit through a wire mesh strainer. Pour the cider from the pot back into the slow cooker.
5. Cover and cook for an additional 15 minutes.

INGREDIENT TIP: If you like tart cider, then use a more sour apple, like Granny Smith; if you like sweet cider, go with a sweeter variety, like Golden Delicious.

PER SERVING (1 CUP) Calories: 60; Total Fat: 0g; Saturated Fat: 0g; Cholesterol: 0mg; Sodium: 1mg; Potassium: 94mg; Carbs: 16g; Fiber: 2g; Protein: 0g

Granola

MAKES 4 CUPS • **PREP TIME:** 15 MINUTES • **COOK TIME:** 5 TO 6 HOURS ON LOW

LOWEST SODIUM

LOW-CHOLESTEROL • VEGETARIAN

Store-bought granola is a huge culprit when it comes to hidden sodium and sugars. Making your own eliminates all the mystery around what's actually in it, and it's usually cheaper, too. This recipe uses regular, old-fashioned oats instead of instant or quick. Feel free to jazz it up by adding in ¼ cup nuts, seeds, or dried unsweetened fruit.

Nonstick cooking spray

2 cups rolled oats (regular or old-fashioned, not instant or quick)

¼ cup nuts, seeds, or dried unsweetened fruit (optional)

2 tablespoons coconut oil, melted

2 tablespoons honey

1 teaspoon pure vanilla extract

2 teaspoons ground cinnamon (or as much or little as desired)

Fresh fruit and berries, for garnish (optional)

1. Spray the slow cooker generously with nonstick cooking spray.
2. Add the oats and nuts, seeds, or dried fruit (if using) to the slow cooker. Stir to mix well.
3. In a medium bowl, whisk the coconut oil with the honey, vanilla, and cinnamon. Pour the mixture into the slow cooker, stirring to make sure all the ingredients are coated.
4. Lay a dish towel between the slow cooker and the lid. This will absorb all the condensation so it won't drip back onto the granola while it cooks, making it soggy.
5. Cover and cook on low for 5 to 6 hours.
6. Using a spatula, transfer the granola to a baking sheet to cool. Serve garnished with fruit and berries (if using).

STORAGE TIP: Store in an airtight container at room temperature or in the refrigerator for up to 2 weeks. You can freeze this granola for up to 2 months.

PER SERVING (1 CUP) Calories: 399; Total Fat: 12g; Saturated Fat: 7g; Cholesterol: 0mg; Sodium: 2mg; Potassium: 347mg; Carbs: 61g; Fiber: 9g; Protein: 13g

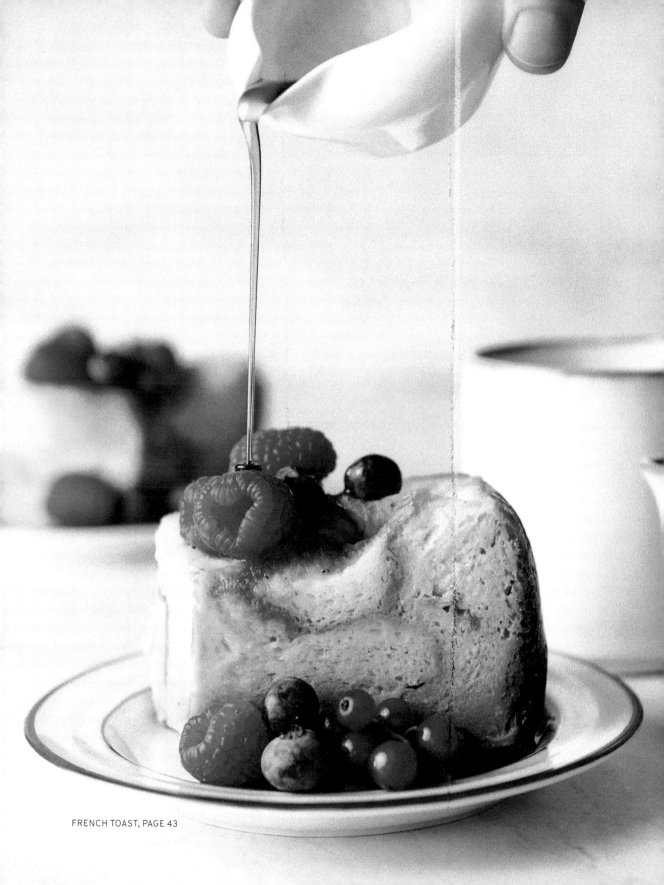

FRENCH TOAST, PAGE 43

Breakfasts

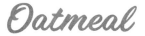

Oatmeal

SERVES 4 • **PREP TIME:** 5 MINUTES • **COOK TIME:** 6 TO 8 HOURS ON LOW

LOWEST SODIUM

ALLERGY-FRIENDLY • LOW-CHOLESTEROL • VEGETARIAN

Oatmeal is the epitome of a heart-friendly, healthy, and hearty breakfast. This recipe uses steel-cut oats, not rolled or instant (the flat grains you typically see in the supermarket for making oatmeal). Steel-cut oats need to cook low and slow, making them perfect for overnight in the slow cooker. You have some leeway in this recipe when it comes to ingredient add-ins. Fruits like apples, bananas, and berries, or even nuts and seeds are healthy additions to this oatmeal. You can stir them in with the rest of the ingredients at the start of cooking or use them as toppings.

Nonstick cooking spray

1 cup steel-cut oats

2½ cups water

2 tablespoons honey (or maple syrup if vegan)

½ teaspoon pure vanilla extract

1 teaspoon ground cinnamon

1. Spray the slow cooker generously with nonstick cooking spray.
2. In the slow cooker, combine the oats, water, honey, vanilla, and cinnamon. Stir to mix well.
3. Cook on low for 6 to 8 hours and serve.

VARIATION: For a creamier oatmeal, use milk or almond milk instead of water.

PER SERVING Calories: 205; Total Fat: 1g; Saturated Fat: 0g; Cholesterol: 0mg; Sodium: 1mg; Potassium: 9mg; Carbs: 38g; Fiber: 5g; Protein: 7g

Protein Oatmeal Bake

SERVES 8 • **PREP TIME:** 5 MINUTES • **COOK TIME:** 6 TO 8 HOURS ON LOW

LOWER SODIUM

VEGETARIAN

Oatmeal is one of the healthiest foods you can eat. As part of a healthy diet, it's been known to lower the risk of heart disease and reduce levels of bad (LDL) cholesterol. Adding your preferred protein powder turns this overnight breakfast meal into the perfect workout fuel.

Nonstick cooking spray

2 cups steel-cut oats

2 teaspoons protein powder

1 teaspoon baking powder

1 teaspoon ground cinnamon

½ teaspoon salt

2 cups almond milk

¼ cup honey

1 ripe banana, mashed

1 large egg

1 tablespoon pure vanilla extract

1. Spray the slow cooker generously with nonstick cooking spray.
2. In a large bowl, mix together the oats, protein powder, baking powder, cinnamon, salt, milk, honey, banana, egg, and vanilla. Pour the mixture into the slow cooker.
3. Cook on low for 6 to 8 hours, or until the oatmeal is set, and serve.

VARIATION: Add your other favorite fruits to this! Apples or berries, in particular, are good additions. Stir them directly into the slow cooker at the start of cooking.

PER SERVING Calories: 245; Total Fat: 4g; Saturated Fat: 1g; Cholesterol: 26mg; Sodium: 194mg; Potassium: 141mg; Carbs: 44g; Fiber: 6g; Protein: 8g

Cheese Grits

SERVES 8 • **PREP TIME:** 5 MINUTES • **COOK TIME:** 6 TO 8 HOURS ON LOW

LOW SODIUM

LOW-CARB • LOW-CHOLESTEROL • VEGETARIAN

Traditionally prepared with lots of cheese and salt, grits aren't necessarily considered a healthy dish. But it's easy to lighten them up without sacrificing flavor. This recipe calls for stone-ground grits, because they're better suited for the long, slow cook. But they can be hard to find, so you can also use quick grits. Just be sure not to use instant grits.

Nonstick cooking spray

1½ cups stone-ground grits

3 cups skim milk or almond milk

3 cups water

1 cup Cheddar cheese, shredded

2 teaspoons ghee (clarified butter)

1 teaspoon salt

½ teaspoon freshly ground black pepper

1. Spray the slow cooker generously with nonstick cooking spray.

2. In the slow cooker, combine the grits, milk, water, cheese, ghee, salt, and pepper. Stir to mix well.

3. Cook on low for 6 to 8 hours.

4. Stir to mix well, and check the consistency. You can cook a bit longer for a thicker consistency, but keep in mind they will thicken as they stand. Once your desired consistency is reached, serve immediately.

VARIATION: You don't have to use Cheddar cheese. Consider mozzarella, provolone, or even Gruyère. Just make sure you use a cheese that melts easily.

PER SERVING Calories: 201; Total Fat: 8g; Saturated Fat: 3g; Cholesterol: 15mg; Sodium: 431mg; Potassium: 54mg; Carbs: 26g; Fiber: 1g; Protein: 6g

French Toast

SERVES 8 • **PREP TIME:** 5 MINUTES • **COOK TIME:** 6 TO 8 HOURS ON LOW

LOW SODIUM

LOW-CARB • VEGETARIAN

This French toast will look like a fluffy bread pudding/soufflé when it's done. To brown the top of the bread, remove the lid but keep the cooker on about 15 minutes before serving. You can serve this with your favorite syrup or, depending on what fruit you use, you might not need syrup at all.

Nonstick cooking spray

1 loaf sliced challah bread

12 large eggs

4 cups low-fat milk

2 teaspoons ground cinnamon

2 tablespoons honey or
  maple syrup

2 teaspoons pure vanilla extract

1. Spray the slow cooker generously with nonstick cooking spray.
2. Layer the bread slices in the bottom of the slow cooker.
3. In a large bowl, whisk together the eggs, milk, cinnamon, honey, and vanilla. Pour the mixture over the bread, making sure all the pieces are soaked.
4. Cook on low for 6 to 8 hours and serve.

VARIATION: Before serving, add fresh fruit, berries, or nuts such as chopped pecans to make this a complete breakfast meal.

PER SERVING Calories: 290; Total Fat: 11g; Saturated Fat: 3g; Cholesterol: 323mg; Sodium: 425mg; Potassium: 432mg; Carbs: 30g; Fiber: 3g; Protein: 20g

Egg White Vegetable Frittata

SERVES 8 TO 12 • **PREP TIME:** 10 MINUTES • **COOK TIME:** 6 TO 8 HOURS ON LOW

LOWER SODIUM

GLUTEN-FREE • LOW-CARB • LOW-CHOLESTEROL • VEGETARIAN

In terms of healthy breakfast recipes, this one nails it. It's low-carb, low-sodium, and packed with protein and vegetables. Load this one up with your favorite veggies. You really can't go wrong here; spinach, kale, mushrooms, tomatoes, and bell peppers all make great additions. If you have fresh herbs, chop them up and toss them in as well.

Nonstick cooking spray

2 cups egg whites (from about 12 large eggs)

1½ cups chopped vegetables (spinach, tomatoes, bell peppers, mushrooms, etc.)

½ cup grated low-fat Cheddar cheese

½ cup low-fat or skim milk

1 garlic clove, minced

¼ cup diced onion

Salt

Freshly ground black pepper

1. Spray the slow cooker generously with nonstick cooking spray.
2. In a large bowl, whisk together the egg whites, vegetables, cheese, milk, garlic, and onion. Season lightly with salt and pepper, and pour into the slow cooker.
3. Cook on low for 6 to 8 hours, or until the eggs are set, and serve.

SUBSTITUTION TIP: If you have a dairy allergy, simply substitute almond milk and omit the cheese, or use a vegan cheese.

PER SERVING Calories: 73; Total Fat: 1g; Saturated Fat: 0g; Cholesterol: 2mg; Sodium: 177mg; Potassium: 198mg; Carbs: 6g; Fiber: 2g; Protein: 10g

Eggs with Green Bell Peppers and Diced Tomatoes

SERVES 12 • **PREP TIME:** 10 MINUTES • **COOK TIME:** 6 TO 8 HOURS ON LOW

LOWER SODIUM

GLUTEN-FREE • LOW-CARB • VEGETARIAN

This is a little bit like Middle Eastern shakshuka—eggs poached in a sauce made from tomatoes, peppers, onions, and cumin. You really can't go wrong here in terms of adding in extra diced vegetables or even meats. All the ingredients cooked together provide a flavorful, hearty breakfast bowl.

Nonstick cooking spray

12 large eggs

¼ cup low-fat milk

1 (28-ounce) can no-salt-added diced tomatoes, drained

1 small onion, diced

1 green bell pepper, seeded and diced

1 teaspoon dried oregano

1 teaspoon ground cumin

½ teaspoon salt

¼ teaspoon freshly ground black pepper

1. Spray the slow cooker generously with nonstick cooking spray.

2. In a large bowl, whisk the eggs until they are thoroughly combined, then mix in the milk, tomatoes, onion, bell pepper, oregano, cumin, salt, and pepper. Pour the mixture into the slow cooker.

3. Cook on low for 6 to 8 hours, or until the eggs are set, and serve.

VARIATION: Add up to ½ pound of your preferred low-sodium cooked and diced meat to this dish.

PER SERVING Calories: 88; Total Fat: 5g; Saturated Fat: 2g; Cholesterol: 212mg; Sodium: 173mg; Potassium: 217mg; Carbs: 4g; Fiber: 1g; Protein: 7g

Breakfast Scramble

SERVES 6 • **PREP TIME:** 5 MINUTES • **COOK TIME:** 4 TO 6 HOURS ON LOW

LOWER SODIUM

GLUTEN-FREE • LOW-CARB

Eggs, your favorite cheese, vegetables, and cooked meat such as Breakfast Sausage (page 48) are the main ingredients in this easy slow cooker recipe. If you want to make this dish big enough to serve more people, you can add up to ½ pound more of your favorite vegetables or meat without having to change anything else in the recipe. You can also wait until after the eggs are cooked, and then stir in some more cooked meat or vegetables.

Nonstick cooking spray

12 large eggs

¾ cup low-fat milk or almond milk

Salt

Freshly ground black pepper

½ pound ground meat (turkey, pork, or beef), cooked

1. Spray the slow cooker generously with nonstick cooking spray.

2. In a large bowl, whisk together the eggs and milk, and season lightly with salt and pepper. Stir in the meat (or any additional add-ins).

3. Cook on low for 4 to 6 hours, or until the eggs are set.

4. Fluff up the egg mixture before serving.

SUBSTITUTION TIP: Grab your favorite vegetables and/or cheeses and leave out the meat to make this a vegetarian dish.

PER SERVING Calories: 230; Total Fat: 13g; Saturated Fat: 5g; Cholesterol: 458mg; Sodium: 206mg; Potassium: 363mg; Carbs: 2g; Fiber: 0g; Protein: 25g

Breakfast Potatoes

SERVES 6 TO 8 • **PREP TIME:** 10 MINUTES • **COOK TIME:** 6 TO 8 HOURS ON LOW

LOW SODIUM

ALLERGY-FRIENDLY • GLUTEN-FREE • LOW-CHOLESTEROL • VEGAN

Restaurant-style breakfast potatoes can easily be made in the slow cooker. While you can use any variety of potato, waxy, hard red or yellow potatoes work best. You can even substitute sweet potatoes. Substitute fresh herbs for dried if you have them, too. If you use fresh herbs, multiply the amount by three. (So, for example, you'd add 1½ teaspoons of fresh rosemary.)

Nonstick cooking spray

2 pounds potatoes, chopped

2 teaspoons extra-virgin olive oil

¼ cup low-sodium
vegetable broth

1 small onion, diced

½ teaspoon dried rosemary

½ teaspoon paprika

½ teaspoon dried thyme

1 teaspoon salt

½ teaspoon freshly ground
black pepper

1. Spray the slow cooker generously with nonstick cooking spray.

2. In a large bowl, combine the potatoes, olive oil, broth, onion, rosemary, paprika, thyme, salt, and pepper. Stir to evenly coat the potatoes, and pour the mixture into the slow cooker.

3. Cook on low for 6 to 8 hours, or until the potatoes are soft, and serve.

VARIATION: If you're a meat-eater, you can stir in 5 or 6 slices of cooked and crumbled low-sodium bacon after the potatoes are done cooking.

PER SERVING Calories: 140; Total Fat: 2g; Saturated Fat: 0g; Cholesterol: 0mg; Sodium: 399mg; Potassium: 660mg; Carbs: 29g; Fiber: 2g; Protein: 4g

Breakfast Sausage

SERVES 8 • **PREP TIME:** 5 MINUTES • **COOK TIME:** 6 TO 8 HOURS ON LOW

LOW SODIUM

ALLERGY-FRIENDLY • GLUTEN-FREE • LOW-CARB

Lean ground meat, along with fresh herbs and seasonings, produces a healthy, homemade breakfast sausage so good you'll never buy store-bought again. No need to spray the slow cooker with nonstick cooking spray; the natural grease from the meat should keep it from sticking. You can also put a circle of aluminum foil or parchment paper in the bottom of the slow cooker for easy cleanup.

1 pound lean ground pork

1 garlic clove, minced

1 teaspoon salt

1 teaspoon dried thyme

½ teaspoon dried oregano

½ teaspoon onion powder

¼ teaspoon freshly ground black pepper

¼ teaspoon paprika

¼ teaspoon ground cinnamon

1. In a large mixing bowl, combine the pork, garlic, salt, thyme, oregano, onion powder, pepper, paprika, and cinnamon.
2. Press the meat mixture evenly into the bottom of the slow cooker.
3. Cook on low for 6 to 8 hours, or until the meat is completely cooked through.
4. Blot any extra grease off the top, if needed, using a paper towel.
5. Transfer the meat to a cutting board, cut the sausage into squares or circles, and serve.

VARIATION: Use your preferred ground meat—pork, chicken, beef, or turkey. Whatever you choose, it goes in raw. Also feel free to switch up the herbs.

PER SERVING Calories: 150; Total Fat: 12g; Saturated Fat: 4g; Cholesterol: 41mg; Sodium: 323mg; Potassium: 169mg; Carbs: 0g; Fiber: 0g; Protein: 10g

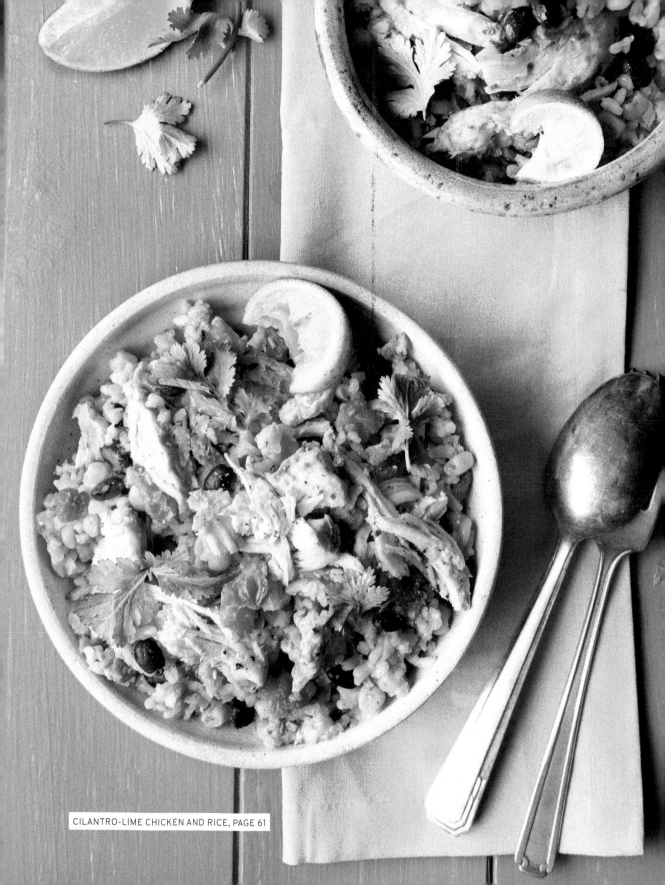

CILANTRO-LIME CHICKEN AND RICE, PAGE 61

Beans and Grains

Cuban Black Beans

SERVES 6 • **PREP TIME:** 10 MINUTES, PLUS OVERNIGHT TO SOAK THE BEANS
COOK TIME: 6 TO 8 HOURS ON LOW

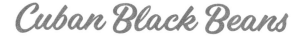

LOWEST SODIUM

ALLERGY-FRIENDLY • GLUTEN-FREE • LOW-CHOLESTEROL • VEGAN

These beans are so hearty and flavorful that they can be served as a main dish. By using dry beans rather than canned, you instantly eliminate a lot of sodium. Plus, they're cheaper. Just be sure to soak your beans overnight. Rinse them in a wire mesh strainer, then pour them into a big bowl and add enough cool water to bring the water level a few inches above the beans.

Nonstick cooking spray

1 pound dry black beans, soaked overnight

3½ cups water

1 large onion, chopped

1 bell pepper, seeded and chopped

1½ teaspoons ground cumin

4 garlic cloves, minced

1 teaspoon dried oregano

Juice of 1 lime

2 dried bay leaves

¼ teaspoon red pepper flakes

¼ cup chopped fresh cilantro

1. Spray the slow cooker generously with nonstick cooking spray.
2. In the slow cooker, combine the beans, water, onion, bell pepper, cumin, garlic, oregano, lime juice, bay leaves, and red pepper flakes. Stir to mix well.
3. Cook on low for 6 to 8 hours.
4. Remove the bay leaves and stir in the cilantro before serving.

VARIATION: If meat is part of your diet, tossing some cooked and crumbled low-sodium bacon in with the beans at the start of cooking is a great way to add a more complex flavor to this recipe.

PER SERVING Calories: 279; Total Fat: 1g; Saturated Fat: 0g; Cholesterol: 0mg; Sodium: 6mg; Potassium: 1,222mg; Carbs: 52g; Fiber: 13g; Protein: 17g

"Refried" Pinto Beans

SERVES 4 • **PREP TIME:** 5 MINUTES, PLUS OVERNIGHT TO SOAK THE BEANS
COOK TIME: 6 TO 8 HOURS ON LOW

LOW SODIUM

ALLERGY-FRIENDLY • GLUTEN-FREE • LOW-CHOLESTEROL • VEGAN

Pinto beans not only contain a lot of nutrients, they're also low in saturated fat and are a good source of protein and fiber. There's nothing "refried" about these pinto beans, but they still have all the flavors of restaurant-style refried beans.

Nonstick cooking spray

½ pound dry pinto beans, soaked overnight

4½ cups water

1 small onion, peeled and quartered

1 jalapeño pepper, stemmed and quartered

2 garlic cloves, minced

½ teaspoon salt

½ teaspoon freshly ground black pepper

½ teaspoon ground cumin

1. Spray the slow cooker generously with nonstick cooking spray.
2. In the slow cooker, combine the beans, water, onion, jalapeño, garlic, salt, pepper, and cumin. Stir to mix well.
3. Cook on low for 6 to 8 hours, or until the beans are tender.
4. Drain the beans through a wire strainer, reserving some of the water for mashing.
5. Using a potato masher or an immersion blender, mash the beans until they reach your desired consistency. Use some of the cooking liquid to thin out the beans, if needed, and serve.

VARIATION: For a bit more flavor, use low-sodium chicken or vegetable broth instead of water.

PER SERVING Calories: 207; Total Fat: 1g; Saturated Fat: 0g; Cholesterol: 0mg; Sodium: 298mg; Potassium: 830mg; Carbs: 38g; Fiber: 9g; Protein: 12g

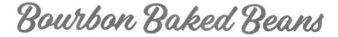

Bourbon Baked Beans

SERVES 8 • **PREP TIME:** 10 MINUTES, PLUS OVERNIGHT TO SOAK THE BEANS
COOK TIME: 6 TO 8 HOURS ON LOW

LOW SODIUM

ALLERGY-FRIENDLY • GLUTEN-FREE • LOW-CHOLESTEROL • VEGAN

Throw the canned baked beans away! Making your own is so much healthier. Again, using dry ingredients eliminates a lot of the sodium content. The combo of bourbon, maple syrup, and ketchup makes for a sweet and savory side dish.

Nonstick cooking spray

1 pound dry great northern beans, soaked overnight

5 cups low-sodium vegetable broth

1 onion, diced

1 bell pepper, seeded and diced

2 garlic cloves, minced

3 tablespoons bourbon

½ cup maple syrup

⅓ cup Ketchup (page 25)

2 teaspoons no-salt-added tomato paste

1 teaspoon ground cumin

1 teaspoon paprika

1 teaspoon salt

½ teaspoon freshly ground black pepper

1. Spray the slow cooker generously with nonstick cooking spray.
2. In the slow cooker, combine the beans, broth, onion, bell pepper, garlic, bourbon, syrup, ketchup, tomato paste, cumin, paprika, salt, and pepper. Stir to mix well.
3. Cook on low for 6 to 8 hours.
4. Stir before serving.

VARIATION: Add ½ pound of low-sodium cooked, crumbled bacon to this recipe at the start of the cook time.

PER SERVING Calories: 287; Total Fat: 1g; Saturated Fat: 0g; Cholesterol: 0mg; Sodium: 374mg; Potassium: 1,052mg; Carbs: 54g; Fiber: 10g; Protein: 16g

Italian Chickpeas

SERVES 6 • **PREP TIME:** 5 MINUTES, PLUS OVERNIGHT TO SOAK THE BEANS
COOK TIME: 4 TO 6 HOURS ON LOW

LOW SODIUM

ALLERGY-FRIENDLY • GLUTEN-FREE • LOW-CHOLESTEROL • VEGAN

Chickpeas are common in Middle Eastern cooking. They're great additions to recipes, but they can also make good stand-alone dishes. When this dish is cooked, it's a bit like a thick stew. Before you soak your chickpeas, sort through them and remove any stones or debris you find.

1 pound dry chickpeas, soaked overnight

1 (28-ounce) can no-salt-added diced tomatoes

1 onion, chopped

1 bell pepper, seeded and chopped

3 garlic cloves, minced

1 teaspoon salt

½ teaspoon freshly ground black pepper

½ teaspoon paprika

½ teaspoon dried basil

½ teaspoon dried oregano

½ teaspoon dried parsley

¼ teaspoon red pepper flakes

1. In the slow cooker, combine the chickpeas, tomatoes and their juices, onion, bell pepper, garlic, salt, pepper, paprika, basil, oregano, parsley, and red pepper flakes. Stir to mix well.

2. Cook on low for 4 to 6 hours, or until the chickpeas are tender, and serve.

VARIATION: Serve this dish over rice or pasta, or even in a tortilla or pita.

PER SERVING Calories: 289; Total Fat: 5g; Saturated Fat: 0g; Cholesterol: 0mg; Sodium: 407mg; Potassium: 733mg; Carbs: 49g; Fiber: 14g; Protein: 15g

Sweet and Spicy Chickpeas

SERVES 8 • **PREP TIME:** 5 MINUTES, PLUS OVERNIGHT TO SOAK THE BEANS
COOK TIME: 4 TO 6 HOURS ON LOW

LOW SODIUM

LOW-CHOLESTEROL • VEGETARIAN

A homemade sweet and spicy sauce is the perfect accompaniment to chickpeas. This savory dish can be served as an appetizer, side dish, or even a main. You can use whatever potatoes you prefer, red-skin potatoes or brown. You can even use chopped sweet potatoes in this recipe.

2 pounds dry chickpeas, soaked overnight

2 bell peppers, seeded and chopped

1 onion, chopped

1 pound potatoes, peeled and chopped

¾ cup honey

⅓ cup sriracha sauce

2 tablespoons low-sodium soy sauce or tamari

2 garlic cloves, minced

1 teaspoon dried basil

1. In the slow cooker, combine the chickpeas, bell peppers, onion, and potatoes.

2. In a medium bowl, mix together the honey, sriracha, soy sauce, garlic, and basil. Pour the sauce into the slow cooker, and stir to mix well.

3. Cook on low for 4 to 6 hours and serve.

SUBSTITUTION TIP: Use tamari instead of soy sauce to make this gluten-free. To make it vegan, add maple syrup rather than honey.

PER SERVING Calories: 570; Total Fat: 7g; Saturated Fat: 1g; Cholesterol: 0mg; Sodium: 412mg; Potassium: 1,343mg; Carbs: 109g; Fiber: 21g; Protein: 24g

Mediterranean Chickpeas and Brown Rice

SERVES 4 • **PREP TIME:** 10 MINUTES • **COOK TIME:** 4 TO 6 HOURS ON LOW

LOW SODIUM

ALLERGY-FRIENDLY • GLUTEN-FREE • LOW-CHOLESTEROL • VEGAN

This recipe is so versatile. You can serve it warm or cold, by itself, as a main dish, or as a side dish. It's vegan this way, but you can also toss in some cooked meat or a few chopped hardboiled eggs at the end for even more protein, or sprinkle 1 cup of shredded cheese over the top before cooking. Be sure to use a low-fat cheese that melts easily, like mozzarella or Gruyère.

Nonstick cooking spray

1 (15-ounce) can chickpeas, drained and rinsed

1 cup uncooked brown rice

2½ cups low-sodium vegetable broth

3 garlic cloves, minced

Juice of 1 lemon

1 tablespoon extra-virgin olive oil

1 teaspoon dried oregano

1 teaspoon paprika

1 teaspoon ground coriander

1 teaspoon ground cumin

1 teaspoon curry powder

1 teaspoon chili powder

½ teaspoon salt

¼ teaspoon freshly ground black pepper

1. Spray the slow cooker generously with nonstick cooking spray.
2. In the slow cooker, combine the chickpeas, rice, broth, garlic, lemon juice, olive oil, oregano, paprika, coriander, cumin, curry powder, chili powder, salt, and pepper. Stir to mix well.
3. Cook on low for 4 to 6 hours, or until the rice is tender, and serve.

VARIATION: To kick this up a couple of notches and add some heat, stir in ½ teaspoon (or more) of red pepper flakes at the start of cooking.

PER SERVING Calories: 372; Total Fat: 8g; Saturated Fat: 1g; Cholesterol: 0mg; Sodium: 353mg; Potassium: 580mg; Carbs: 62g; Fiber: 9g; Protein: 14g

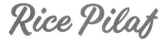

Rice Pilaf

SERVES 4 • PREP TIME: 5 MINUTES **• COOK TIME:** 4 TO 6 HOURS ON LOW

LOW SODIUM

ALLERGY-FRIENDLY • GLUTEN-FREE • LOW-CHOLESTEROL • VEGAN

This rice pilaf is simple yet satisfying—and fairly foolproof. Rice pilaf is a nice, healthy side dish you can serve with just about anything: poultry, red meat, or seafood. One of the main differences between short-grain and long-grain rice is the amount of starch. Short-grain has more starch, which makes it sticky when it cooks (that's why it's used for sushi). Long-grain has less starch and is often used in pilafs.

Nonstick cooking spray

1 cup uncooked long-grain brown rice

2¼ cups low-sodium vegetable broth

1 teaspoon extra-virgin olive oil

½ teaspoon salt

⅛ teaspoon freshly ground black pepper

1. Spray the slow cooker generously with nonstick cooking spray.
2. In the slow cooker, combine the rice, broth, olive oil, salt, and pepper. Stir to mix well.
3. Cook on low for 4 to 6 hours and serve.

VARIATION: Add some protein by tossing a handful of chopped nuts into the slow cooker with the rest of the ingredients. Pecans, walnuts, or almonds are good choices, or try shelled sunflower or pumpkin seeds.

PER SERVING Calories: 203; Total Fat: 3g; Saturated Fat: 1g; Cholesterol: 0mg; Sodium: 334mg; Potassium: 218mg; Carbs: 37g; Fiber: 2g; Protein: 6g

Wild Rice and Mushroom Casserole

SERVES 4 • **PREP TIME:** 10 MINUTES • **COOK TIME:** 5 TO 7 HOURS ON LOW

LOW SODIUM

ALLERGY-FRIENDLY • GLUTEN-FREE • LOW-CARB • LOW-CHOLESTEROL

Wild rice is high in protein and fiber, and low in fat. It cooks directly in the slow cooker with mushrooms, broth, and seasonings in this delicious casserole. You can use whatever type of mushrooms you love—button, cremini, baby portobellos, or a combination.

Nonstick cooking spray

1 pound mushrooms, sliced

¾ cup uncooked wild rice

1½ cups low-sodium chicken broth

1 onion, finely chopped

¼ teaspoon dried thyme

¼ teaspoon dried basil

½ teaspoon salt

½ teaspoon freshly ground black pepper

2 tablespoons chopped fresh parsley

1. Spray the slow cooker generously with nonstick cooking spray.
2. In the slow cooker, combine the mushrooms, rice, broth, onion, thyme, basil, salt, and pepper. Stir to mix well.
3. Cook on low for 5 to 7 hours, or until the rice is tender.
4. Top with fresh parsley and serve.

VARIATION: Like cheese? Sprinkle about ½ cup of shredded mozzarella or Gruyère cheese over the top during the last 30 minutes of cook time. To make this vegan, switch the chicken broth for low-sodium vegetable broth.

PER SERVING Calories: 154; Total Fat: 1g; Saturated Fat: 0g; Cholesterol: 0mg; Sodium: 327mg; Potassium: 602mg; Carbs: 29g; Fiber: 3g; Protein: 10g

Rice with Chicken and Asparagus

SERVES 4 • **PREP TIME:** 5 MINUTES • **COOK TIME:** 5 TO 7 HOURS ON LOW

LOW SODIUM

ALLERGY-FRIENDLY • GLUTEN-FREE

One-pot meals are meant to be easy, but that doesn't mean they also have to be boring. While this recipe calls for brown rice, you can use white if you prefer. You can also use chicken thighs or breasts or a mixture.

Nonstick cooking spray

1 pound boneless, skinless chicken breasts or thighs

1 cup uncooked brown rice

2½ cups water

1 pound asparagus, cut into 1-inch pieces

2 garlic cloves, minced

Juice of 2 limes

1 teaspoon ground cumin

½ teaspoon salt

½ teaspoon freshly ground black pepper

1. Spray the slow cooker generously with nonstick cooking spray.
2. In the slow cooker, combine the chicken, rice, water, asparagus, garlic, lime juice, cumin, salt, and pepper. Stir to mix well.
3. Cook on low for 5 to 7 hours, or until the rice is tender, and serve.

VARIATION: If you can't find or don't like asparagus, substitute green beans.

PER SERVING Calories: 321; Total Fat: 3g; Saturated Fat: 1g; Cholesterol: 66mg; Sodium: 370mg; Potassium: 627mg; Carbs: 41g; Fiber: 4g; Protein: 32g

Cilantro-Lime Chicken and Rice

SERVES 6 • **PREP TIME:** 10 MINUTES • **COOK TIME:** 5 TO 7 HOURS ON LOW

LOW SODIUM

ALLERGY-FRIENDLY

Cilantro is the leafy part of the same herb from which we get coriander. The little coriander seeds are actually the fruit of the plant. Fresh coriander leaves have a bright, citrusy flavor that you can't get from parsley or any other leafy green herb. Because heat takes away the bright flavor, cilantro is usually added to a dish after it is cooked.

Nonstick cooking spray

1 pound boneless, skinless chicken breasts or thighs

2 cups uncooked brown rice

4 cups water

1 (15-ounce) can no-salt-added diced tomatoes

1 (15-ounce) can black beans, drained and rinsed

1 (15-ounce) can corn, drained and rinsed

2 garlic cloves, minced

Juice of 2 limes

1 teaspoon ground cumin

1 teaspoon salt

½ teaspoon freshly ground black pepper

½ teaspoon dried oregano

½ cup chopped fresh cilantro

1. Spray the slow cooker generously with nonstick cooking spray.
2. In the slow cooker, combine the chicken, rice, water, tomatoes and their juices, beans, corn, garlic, lime juice, cumin, salt, pepper, and oregano. Stir to mix well.
3. Cook on low for 5 to 7 hours, or until the rice is tender.
4. Sprinkle with fresh cilantro before serving.

SUBSTITUTION TIP: To make this meal vegan, leave out the chicken and add ½ pound of dry black beans that have been soaked overnight.

PER SERVING Calories: 432; Total Fat: 3g; Saturated Fat: 1g; Cholesterol: 44mg; Sodium: 448mg; Potassium: 815mg; Carbs: 72g; Fiber: 7g; Protein: 29g

Indian Spiced Brown Rice with Ground Lamb

SERVES 6 • **PREP TIME:** 5 MINUTES • **COOK TIME:** 4 TO 6 HOURS ON LOW

LOWEST SODIUM

ALLERGY-FRIENDLY • GLUTEN-FREE

Curry powder or garam masala? They're both Indian spice blends. Curry powder is a blend of 20 herbs and spices. Garam masala is also a blend of spices, but with less heat. Whichever you choose, it will not only provide a flavorful kick to this dish, but the aroma will have your entire house smelling amazing.

1 cup uncooked brown rice

2 cups low-sodium chicken broth

1 cup Marinara Sauce (page 30)

1 onion, chopped

3 garlic cloves, minced

2 teaspoons curry powder or garam masala

2 teaspoons ground cumin

2 teaspoons ground ginger

2 teaspoons ground turmeric

1 teaspoon ground coriander

½ teaspoon ground cayenne pepper

1 pound ground lamb, cooked

1. In the slow cooker, combine the rice, broth, marinara sauce, onion, garlic, curry powder, cumin, ginger, turmeric, coriander, and cayenne pepper. Stir to mix well.
2. Cook on low for 4 to 6 hours.
3. Stir in the ground lamb and serve.

VARIATION: If you're not a fan of lamb, substitute the same amount of cooked ground beef, chicken, turkey, or pork.

PER SERVING Calories: 325; Total Fat: 13g; Saturated Fat: 5g; Cholesterol: 51mg; Sodium: 83mg; Potassium: 505mg; Carbs: 33g; Fiber: 3g; Protein: 18g

Barley and Chickpea Risotto

SERVES 4 • **PREP TIME:** 5 MINUTES • **COOK TIME:** 4 TO 6 HOURS ON LOW

LOW SODIUM

LOW-CHOLESTEROL • VEGETARIAN

Both barley and chickpeas are high in fiber, improve digestion, and help fight heart disease. Combining the two is a win-win. You'd never think risotto could be so creamy, easy, and healthy, all at the same time.

Nonstick cooking spray

1½ cups uncooked barley, rinsed

1 (15-ounce) can chickpeas, drained and rinsed

3 cups water

2 garlic cloves, minced

1 onion, minced

1 teaspoon salt

½ teaspoon dried rosemary

½ teaspoon freshly ground black pepper

¼ cup grated Parmesan cheese

¼ cup chopped fresh parsley

1. Spray the slow cooker generously with nonstick cooking spray.
2. In the slow cooker, combine the barley, chickpeas, water, garlic, onion, salt, rosemary, pepper, and cheese. Stir to mix well.
3. Cook on low for 4 to 6 hours.
4. Top with fresh parsley before serving.

COOKING TIP: For more flavor, use low-sodium broth instead of water or a combo of the two.

PER SERVING Calories: 445; Total Fat: 5g; Saturated Fat: 2g; Cholesterol: 6mg; Sodium: 416mg; Potassium: 511mg; Carbs: 83g; Fiber: 18g; Protein: 17g

Italian-Style Barley Casserole

SERVES 4 • **PREP TIME:** 10 MINUTES • **COOK TIME:** 5 TO 7 HOURS ON LOW

LOW SODIUM

LOW-CHOLESTEROL • VEGAN

Italian seasonings, olives, and artichokes elevate this basic barley casserole. Use this recipe as a guideline, and start experimenting. Switch up the vegetables, the herbs, even the grain for several different takes on the same dish.

Nonstick cooking spray

1 cup uncooked barley, rinsed

2½ cups water

1 onion, chopped

1 ounce pitted and sliced black olives

1 (6-ounce) can water-packed whole artichokes, drained and quartered

1 cup Marinara Sauce (page 30)

3 garlic cloves, minced

½ teaspoon salt

½ teaspoon freshly ground black pepper

½ teaspoon paprika

½ teaspoon dried basil

½ teaspoon dried oregano

½ teaspoon dried parsley

¼ teaspoon red pepper flakes

1. Spray the slow cooker generously with nonstick cooking spray.
2. In the slow cooker, combine the barley, water, onion, olives, artichokes, marinara sauce, garlic, salt, pepper, paprika, basil, oregano, parsley, and red pepper flakes. Stir to mix well.
3. Cook on low for 5 to 7 hours, or until the barley is tender, and serve.

VARIATION: If you're not vegetarian, this is a great recipe for using some leftover meat, such as chicken breasts. Stir in ½ pound of cut-up cooked meat at the beginning of the cook time.

PER SERVING Calories: 292; Total Fat: 6g; Saturated Fat: 1g; Cholesterol: 1mg; Sodium: 398mg; Potassium: 389mg; Carbs: 56g; Fiber: 12g; Protein: 8g

Beef and Barley Casserole

SERVES 4 • **PREP TIME:** 10 MINUTES • **COOK TIME:** 5 TO 7 HOURS ON LOW

LOW SODIUM

This barley casserole is high-fiber and hearty but also very simple, using just a few ingredients. The barley cooks directly in the slow cooker along with everything else, absorbing all the flavors, making this dish as delicious as it is easy.

Nonstick cooking spray

⅔ cup uncooked barley

1 pound beef stew meat, cut into chunks

1½ cups water

1 onion, chopped

3 carrots, chopped

2 celery stalks, chopped

2 tablespoons low-sodium soy sauce or tamari

1 tablespoon honey

Freshly ground black pepper

1. Spray the slow cooker generously with nonstick cooking spray.
2. In the slow cooker, combine the barley, stew meat, water, onion, carrots, celery, soy sauce, and honey, and season lightly with pepper.
3. Cook on low for 5 to 7 hours, or until the barley is tender and all the water is absorbed, and serve.

VARIATION: Swap ground beef or even ground turkey for the stew meat.

PER SERVING Calories: 318; Total Fat: 6g; Saturated Fat: 2g; Cholesterol: 43mg; Sodium: 377mg; Potassium: 721mg; Carbs: 37g; Fiber: 7g; Protein: 29g

Coconut Quinoa Curry

SERVES 6 • **PREP TIME:** 10 MINUTES • **COOK TIME:** 6 TO 8 HOURS ON LOW

LOW SODIUM

LOW-CARB • LOW-CHOLESTEROL • VEGETARIAN

Packed with flavor, this coconut curry will give you your Thai food fix. Quinoa is a seed and is gluten-free. Rinse the quinoa before cooking to remove the natural coating, which can make it taste bitter or soapy.

1 (15-ounce) can full-fat coconut milk

1 cup Coconut-Curry Sauce (page 32)

1 (15-ounce) can no-salt-added diced tomatoes

1 cup uncooked quinoa, rinsed

1 small onion, chopped

2 garlic cloves, minced

1 tablespoon low-sodium soy sauce (or tamari if gluten-free)

2 teaspoons curry powder

1 teaspoon ground ginger

½ teaspoon salt

½ teaspoon freshly ground black pepper

¼ teaspoon red pepper flakes

1. In the slow cooker, combine the coconut milk, curry sauce, tomatoes and their juices, quinoa, onion, garlic, soy sauce, curry powder, ginger, salt, pepper, and red pepper flakes. Stir to mix well.

2. Cook on low for 6 to 8 hours and serve.

VARIATION: If you don't have or don't like quinoa, you can substitute 1 cup of brown rice instead.

PER SERVING Calories: 445; Total Fat: 32g; Saturated Fat: 27g; Cholesterol: 0mg; Sodium: 358mg; Potassium: 652mg; Carbs: 28g; Fiber: 3g; Protein: 9g

Enchilada Quinoa Bake

SERVES 4 • **PREP TIME:** 10 MINUTES • **COOK TIME:** 5 HOURS 30 MINUTES
TO 7 HOURS 30 MINUTES ON LOW

LOW SODIUM

LOW-CHOLESTEROL • VEGETARIAN

Enchilada flavors slow cook with quinoa in this super easy casserole that's a rich source of fiber and protein. The sky is the limit when it comes to the toppings for this quinoa bake; you can add tomatoes, avocado, green onions, or anything else you can think of to your bowl after this meal is done cooking.

Nonstick cooking spray

1 cup uncooked quinoa, rinsed

1½ cups low-sodium
  vegetable broth

1 cup Enchilada Sauce (page 28)

1 (15-ounce) can black beans,
  drained and rinsed

1 (15-ounce) can corn, drained
  and rinsed

1 cup Marinara Sauce (page 30)

1 onion, chopped

1 bell pepper, seeded
  and chopped

2 garlic cloves, minced

2 tablespoons chili powder

1½ teaspoons ground cumin

½ teaspoon salt

½ teaspoon freshly ground
  black pepper

1 cup low-fat Cheddar cheese

¼ cup chopped fresh cilantro

1. Spray the slow cooker generously with nonstick cooking spray.
2. In the slow cooker, combine the quinoa, broth, enchilada sauce, beans, corn, marinara sauce, onion, bell pepper, garlic, chili powder, cumin, salt, and pepper. Stir to mix well.
3. Cook on low for 5 to 7 hours.
4. Add the cheese and cook another 30 minutes, or until the cheese is melted.
5. Sprinkle with cilantro just before serving.

SUBSTITUTION TIP: This is a vegetarian dish, but you can stir in ½ pound of any uncooked ground meat at the beginning of the cook time. Or go vegan and just leave out the cheese.

PER SERVING Calories: 459; Total Fat: 10g; Saturated Fat: 1g; Cholesterol: 6mg; Sodium: 490mg; Potassium: 1,125mg; Carbs: 73g; Fiber: 13g; Protein: 23g

Quinoa Turkey Chili

SERVES 6 TO 8 • **PREP TIME:** 5 MINUTES • **COOK TIME:** 6 TO 8 HOURS ON LOW

LOW SODIUM

ALLERGY-FRIENDLY • GLUTEN-FREE

Quinoa is naturally gluten-free and high in fiber and protein. Chili is the ultimate comfort food. Combining the two produces a satisfying high-fiber meal. Serve it with a salad on the side so you get your veggies, too.

1 cup uncooked quinoa

1 pound ground turkey

1 (28-ounce) can no-salt-added crushed tomatoes

1 (10-ounce) can no-salt-added diced tomatoes with green chiles

1 cup Marinara Sauce (page 30)

1 (15-ounce) can red kidney beans, drained and rinsed

1 onion, chopped

3 garlic cloves, minced

2 tablespoons chili powder

½ teaspoon salt

2 teaspoons ground cumin

1½ teaspoons paprika

1 teaspoon dried oregano

1. In the slow cooker, combine the quinoa, turkey, crushed and diced tomatoes and their juices, marinara sauce, beans, onion, garlic, chili powder, salt, cumin, paprika, and oregano. Stir to mix well.

2. Cook on low for 6 to 8 hours and serve.

VARIATION: Looking to add more fiber to your diet? Load this dish up with more beans! Chickpeas or black beans are both good additions.

PER SERVING Calories: 365; Total Fat: 4g; Saturated Fat: 1g; Cholesterol: 41mg; Sodium: 456mg; Potassium: 898mg; Carbs: 52g; Fiber: 13g; Protein: 32g

Creamy Millet with Cauliflower

SERVES 4 • **PREP TIME:** 10 MINUTES • **COOK TIME:** 5 TO 7 HOURS ON LOW

LOW SODIUM

ALLERGY-FRIENDLY • VEGAN

Millet is actually a type of grass seed, and it is very versatile. It can be made creamy like mashed potatoes or it can have the consistency of rice. And like oats, it's high in fiber and heart-healthy. It's also a good source of protein. You can find it in the supermarket, along with the rice and quinoa.

1 cup uncooked millet

1 medium head cauliflower, roughly chopped

5 cups low-sodium vegetable broth

1 medium onion, diced

2 garlic cloves, minced

1 teaspoon salt

¼ teaspoon freshly ground black pepper

¼ cup chopped fresh parsley

1. In the slow cooker, combine the millet, cauliflower, broth, onion, garlic, salt, and pepper. Stir to mix well.
2. Cook on low for 5 to 7 hours.
3. Top with fresh parsley and serve.

COOKING TIP: The cauliflower will be very soft when this is done cooking. You can leave it in chunks or use an immersion blender to mash it up.

PER SERVING Calories: 284; Total Fat: 21g; Saturated Fat: 1g; Cholesterol: 31mg; Sodium: 254mg; Potassium: 602mg; Carbs: 47g; Fiber: 9g; Protein: 15g

Spiced Millet with Kielbasa

SERVES 4 • **PREP TIME:** 5 MINUTES • **COOK TIME:** 6 TO 8 HOURS ON LOW

LOW SODIUM

ALLERGY-FRIENDLY

Millet is rich in iron and vitamin B$_6$. Most people eat millet for breakfast, but paired with kielbasa it creates a hearty slow cooker recipe. Kielbasa, like most cured meats, is usually full of sodium. Be sure to find a low- or reduced-sodium version. Serve this with a side of your favorite vegetables or a simple salad for a delicious, healthy meal.

Nonstick cooking spray

1 cup uncooked millet

2 cups any no-salt-added broth

¾ pound low-sodium kielbasa, cut into 1-inch pieces

2 garlic cloves, minced

1 teaspoon paprika

½ teaspoon salt

½ teaspoon onion powder

½ teaspoon dried thyme

½ teaspoon freshly ground black pepper

¼ teaspoon red pepper flakes

1. Spray the slow cooker generously with nonstick cooking spray.

2. In the slow cooker, combine the millet, broth, kielbasa, garlic, paprika, salt, onion powder, thyme, pepper, and red pepper flakes. Stir to mix well.

3. Cook on low for 6 to 8 hours and serve.

VARIATION: For a different flavor, try substituting a low-sodium pork sausage or my Breakfast Sausage (page 48) in place of the kielbasa.

PER SERVING Calories: 398; Total Fat: 19g; Saturated Fat: 6g; Cholesterol: 76mg; Sodium: 490mg; Potassium: 126mg; Carbs: 53g; Fiber: 5g; Protein: 16g

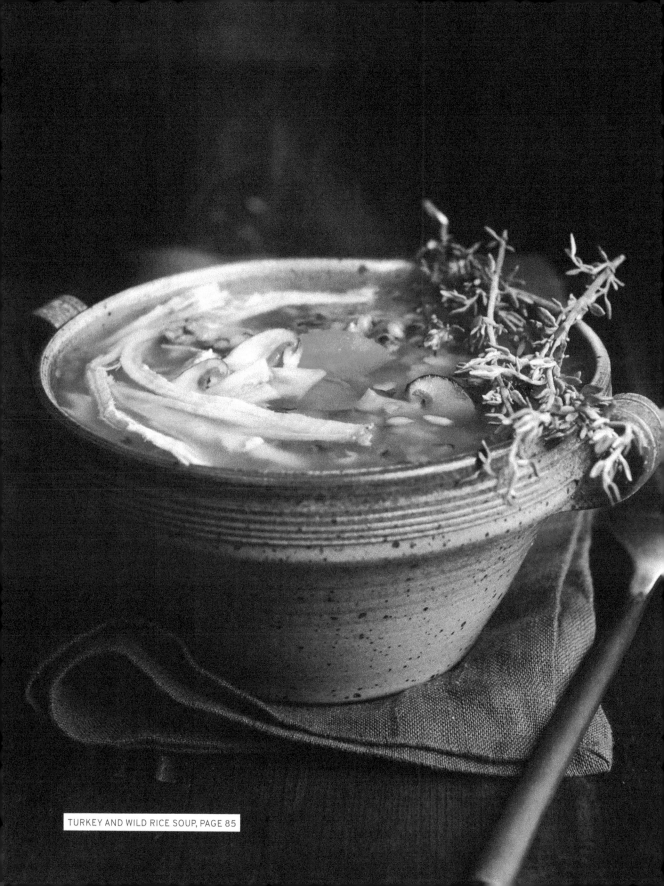

TURKEY AND WILD RICE SOUP, PAGE 85

Soups and Stews

Cauliflower Soup

SERVES 4 • **PREP TIME:** 10 MINUTES • **COOK TIME:** 3 TO 4 HOURS ON LOW

LOW SODIUM

GLUTEN-FREE • LOW-CHOLESTEROL • VEGAN

This basic cauliflower soup is super simple and can even be used as a base for other soups or casseroles. For example, replace canned cream of mushroom soup with a couple cups of this soup when making green bean casserole. This version is vegan, but you can also use chicken broth.

1 head cauliflower, chopped

2 garlic cloves, minced

1 pound potatoes, peeled and roughly chopped

1 large onion, chopped

2 cups almond milk

2 cups low-sodium vegetable broth

½ teaspoon salt

¼ teaspoon freshly ground black pepper

1. In the slow cooker, combine the cauliflower, garlic, potatoes, onion, almond milk, broth, salt, and pepper. Stir to mix well.
2. Cook on low for 3 to 4 hours and serve.

VARIATION: For a thicker, creamier soup, use 1½ cups of almond milk instead of 2.

PER SERVING Calories: 154; Total Fat: 2g; Saturated Fat: 0g; Cholesterol: 0mg; Sodium: 367mg; Potassium: 1,045mg; Carbs: 31g; Fiber: 8g; Protein: 7g

Carrot and Ginger Soup

SERVES 4 • **PREP TIME:** 5 MINUTES • **COOK TIME:** 3 TO 4 HOURS ON LOW

LOW SODIUM

ALLERGY-FRIENDLY • GLUTEN-FREE • LOW-CARB • LOW-CHOLESTEROL • VEGAN

This soup is full of healthy ingredients. Carrots can reduce cholesterol and lower the risk of heart attacks, while ginger is one of the oldest spices around and has long been a fixture in herbal medicine because it aids the immune and digestive systems and relieves pains and nausea. For all that goodness, you'll be surprised how easy it is to make this soup.

2 pounds carrots, peeled and chopped

2 cups water

2 cups low-sodium vegetable broth

1 onion, chopped

1 tablespoon ground ginger

½ teaspoon salt

Fresh parsley, for garnish

1. In the slow cooker, combine the carrots, water, broth, onion, ginger, and salt. Stir to mix well.

2. Cook on low for 3 to 4 hours.

3. Using an immersion blender, blend the soup directly in the slow cooker until it reaches your desired consistency, or carefully transfer to a blender and blend in batches.

4. Garnish with fresh parsley just before serving.

VARIATION: For a creamier version, use coconut milk (full-fat or light) instead of some or all of the broth.

PER SERVING Calories: 116; Total Fat: 0g; Saturated Fat: 0g; Cholesterol: 0mg; Sodium: 383mg; Potassium: 783mg; Carbs: 26g; Fiber: 6g; Protein: 3g

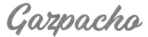

Gazpacho

SERVES 4 • **PREP TIME:** 10 MINUTES • **COOK TIME:** 3 TO 4 HOURS ON LOW

LOW SODIUM

ALLERGY-FRIENDLY • GLUTEN-FREE • LOW-CARB • LOW-CHOLESTEROL • VEGAN

Gazpacho isn't usually associated with the slow cooker because it is served cold—and, typically, raw. But cooking the tomatoes first helps our bodies break down the plant cell walls, enabling us to better absorb the nutrients. Fresh tomatoes and herbs bring a brightness to this recipe that you don't get when you use canned and dried ingredients. The best part is that the tomatoes don't need to be blanched and peeled first.

3 pounds Roma
  tomatoes, chopped

2 tablespoons extra-virgin
  olive oil

¼ cup red wine vinegar

1 cucumber, peeled and chopped

1 onion, chopped

1 bell pepper, seeded
  and chopped

2 garlic cloves, minced

½ teaspoon salt

½ teaspoon ground cumin

¼ teaspoon freshly ground
  black pepper

¼ cup chopped fresh basil

1. In the slow cooker, combine the tomatoes, olive oil, vinegar, cucumber, onion, bell pepper, garlic, salt, cumin, and pepper. Stir to mix well.

2. Cook on low for 3 to 4 hours, then allow to cool completely.

3. Using an immersion blender, blend the gazpacho directly in the slow cooker until it reaches your desired consistency, or carefully transfer to a blender and blend in batches.

4. Top with fresh basil and serve.

STORAGE TIP: Keep any leftovers in the refrigerator for up to 5 days. You can also freeze this gazpacho for up to 2 months.

PER SERVING Calories: 160; Total Fat: 8g; Saturated Fat: 1g; Cholesterol: 0mg; Sodium: 313mg; Potassium: 1,041mg; Carbs: 22g; Fiber: 6g; Protein: 4g

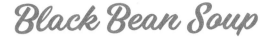

Black Bean Soup

SERVES 4 TO 6 • **PREP TIME:** 5 MINUTES, PLUS OVERNIGHT TO SOAK THE BEANS
COOK TIME: 6 TO 8 HOURS ON LOW

LOW SODIUM

ALLERGY-FRIENDLY • GLUTEN-FREE • LOW-CHOLESTEROL • VEGAN

Black beans are packed with fiber, and when you cook them yourself, they're low-sodium as well. While this soup might look basic, the flavors are anything but. When it's done cooking, mash some of the beans in the slow cooker using the back of a large spoon. This will enhance the flavor.

1 pound dry black beans, soaked overnight

6 cups low-sodium vegetable broth

1 (14.5-ounce) can no-salt-added diced tomatoes

2 bell peppers, seeded and diced

1 onion, diced

3 garlic cloves, minced

1 tablespoon ground cumin

2 teaspoons dried oregano

2 teaspoons paprika

1 teaspoon chili powder

½ teaspoon salt

2 dried bay leaves

1. In the slow cooker, combine the beans, broth, tomatoes and their juices, bell peppers, onion, garlic, cumin, oregano, paprika, chili powder, salt, and bay leaves. Stir to mix well.

2. Cook on low for 6 to 8 hours.

3. Remove the bay leaves before serving.

COOKING TIP: Just before you serve it, top this soup with any or all of these: chopped cilantro, avocado, minced green onions, low-fat grated cheese, and/or low-fat sour cream.

PER SERVING Calories: 464; Total Fat: 3g; Saturated Fat: 1g; Cholesterol: 0mg; Sodium: 423mg; Potassium: 2,238mg; Carbs: 87g; Fiber: 21g; Protein: 27g

Vegetable Minestrone

SERVES 12 • **PREP TIME:** 10 MINUTES • **COOK TIME:** 4 HOURS 15 MINUTES
TO 6 HOURS 30 MINUTES ON LOW

LOWER SODIUM

LOW-CHOLESTEROL • VEGAN

This soup is packed with vegetables, which tend to be naturally low in sodium. The base of this minestrone recipe is just broth, vegetables, and pasta. You can use whatever pasta you prefer—whole-wheat or white. Whole-wheat will make a heartier soup, though, with more fiber.

1 (28-ounce) can no-salt-added diced tomatoes

1 (15-ounce) can no-salt-added crushed tomatoes

6 cups low-sodium vegetable broth

1 (15-ounce) can red kidney beans, drained and rinsed

1 (15-ounce) can great northern beans, drained and rinsed

3 celery stalks, finely chopped

3 carrots, finely chopped

1 medium onion, diced

4 garlic cloves, minced

½ pound green beans, trimmed and cut into 1-inch pieces

2 zucchini, sliced

1 tablespoon Homemade Italian Blend (page 9)

1 teaspoon salt

½ teaspoon freshly ground black pepper

¼ teaspoon ground cumin

2 dried bay leaves

8 ounces uncooked pasta

Fresh parsley, for garnish

1. In the slow cooker, combine the diced and crushed tomatoes with their juices, broth, kidney and great northern beans, celery, carrots, onion, garlic, green beans, zucchini, Italian blend, salt, pepper, cumin, and bay leaves. Stir to mix well.

2. Cook on low for 4 to 6 hours

3. Add the pasta and cook for an additional 15 to 30 minutes, or until the pasta is tender.

4. Remove the bay leaves and sprinkle with parsley just before serving.

SUBSTITUTION TIP: Add even more fiber and make this dish gluten-free and allergy-friendly by using a lentil- or quinoa-based pasta.

PER SERVING Calories: 203; Total Fat: 1g; Saturated Fat: 0g; Cholesterol: 0mg; Sodium: 245mg; Potassium: 647mg; Carbs: 40g; Fiber: 8g; Protein: 11g

Chinese Hot and Sour Soup

SERVES 4 • **PREP TIME:** 10 MINUTES • **COOK TIME:** 3 TO 5 HOURS ON LOW

LOW SODIUM

LOW-CARB • LOW-CHOLESTEROL • VEGAN

This traditional Chinese soup takes its heat from the red pepper flakes and the sour from the rice vinegar. The two flavors complement each other in a wonderful way. While the recipe is vegan, and tofu already gives you lots of protein, you can stir in ½ pound of uncooked meat at the start of the cook time. You can also add cooked ramen noodles—or cooked rice noodles, to keep it gluten-free.

8 ounces firm tofu, cut into
  ½-inch cubes

8 cups low-sodium
  vegetable broth

8 ounces mushrooms, sliced

3 green onions, sliced

3 garlic cloves, minced

2 tablespoons low-sodium soy
  sauce (or tamari if gluten-free)

2 tablespoons rice vinegar

1½ teaspoons ground ginger

1 teaspoon sesame oil

¼ teaspoon salt

¼ teaspoon freshly ground
  black pepper

⅛ teaspoon red pepper flakes

1. In the slow cooker, combine the tofu, broth, mushrooms, green onions, garlic, soy sauce, vinegar, ginger, sesame oil, salt, pepper, and red pepper flakes. Stir to mix well.

2. Cook on low for 3 to 5 hours and serve.

VARIATION: American versions of this soup add a thickening agent like cornstarch. Stir in 3 tablespoons, dissolved in a little water or stock, at the end of cooking.

PER SERVING Calories: 96; Total Fat: 3g; Saturated Fat: 0g; Cholesterol: 0mg; Sodium: 487mg; Potassium: 482mg; Carbs: 10g; Fiber: 1g; Protein: 7g

Green Curry Vegetable Soup

SERVES 4 • **PREP TIME:** 10 MINUTES • **COOK TIME:** 3 TO 4 HOURS ON LOW

LOW SODIUM

LOW-CHOLESTEROL • VEGETARIAN

This recipe calls for a store-bought green curry paste. You should be able to find it in the ethnic foods or Asian foods aisle of your local grocery store. As always, check the ingredients to be sure the curry is made from all-natural ingredients and is low in sodium.

2 cups Coconut-Curry Sauce (page 32)

2 cups water

2 tablespoons green curry paste

1 onion, chopped

1 red bell pepper, seeded and diced

2 zucchini or other summer squash, chopped

½ pound potato or sweet potato, peeled and chopped

1 (8-ounce) can bamboo shoots, drained and rinsed

½ pound green beans, trimmed and cut into 1-inch pieces

1 Asian eggplant, peeled and chopped

1 tablespoon low-sodium soy sauce (or tamari if gluten-free)

1 tablespoon honey

¼ cup chopped fresh basil

1. In the slow cooker, combine the curry sauce, water, curry paste, onion, bell pepper, zucchini, potato, bamboo shoots, green beans, eggplant, soy sauce, honey, and basil. Stir to mix well.

2. Cook on low for 3 to 4 hours and serve.

INGREDIENT TIP: An Asian eggplant may differ from an American one (they're longer, thinner, and less bitter) but it shares the same nutritional benefits. Eggplants are low in saturated fat and sodium and a good source of dietary fiber.

PER SERVING Calories: 390; Total Fat: 25g; Saturated Fat: 20g; Cholesterol: 0mg; Sodium: 443mg; Potassium: 1,426mg; Carbs: 42g; Fiber: 11g; Protein: 10g

Salmon Chowder with Fresh Herbs

SERVES 4 • **PREP TIME:** 10 MINUTES • **COOK TIME:** 3 TO 4 HOURS ON LOW

LOW SODIUM

LOW-CARB

This salmon chowder cooks faster than the usual slow cooker recipe, because fish cooks up so much faster than meat. That means it's not a recipe for which you can throw everything in the pot, go off to work for the day, and come home to a finished dish. But that's not necessarily a bad thing. Because it takes less time, you can be a little more spontaneous about deciding to cook this creamy chowder.

1½ pounds salmon fillets, skinned and cut into 1-inch pieces

5 cups water

3 carrots, peeled and chopped

2 celery stalks, chopped

1 (15-ounce) can corn, drained and rinsed

1 teaspoon Dijon mustard

½ teaspoon salt

1½ tablespoons fresh thyme

1½ tablespoons fresh dill

1. In the slow cooker, combine the salmon, water, carrots, celery, corn, mustard, salt, thyme, and dill. Stir to mix well.
2. Cook on low for 3 to 4 hours and serve.

COOKING TIP: This creamy chowder uses fresh herbs, which add more flavor and a nice aroma, too. If you can't find fresh herbs, you can use dry. Just be sure to use the proper measurement conversion—three times more fresh herbs than dry.

PER SERVING Calories: 288; Total Fat: 7g; Saturated Fat: 1g; Cholesterol: 37mg; Sodium: 397mg; Potassium: 747mg; Carbs: 27g; Fiber: 4g; Protein: 20g

Seafood Chowder

SERVES 4 • **PREP TIME:** 5 MINUTES • **COOK TIME:** 3 HOURS 15 MINUTES
TO 4 HOURS 20 MINUTES ON LOW

LOW SODIUM

Seafood chowder is typically made with milk or cream. To keep this chowder as healthy as possible, I eliminated the cream and used fat-free half-and-half instead. It's still thick and creamy, but without all the fat and cholesterol.

4 cups water

1 cup fat-free half-and-half

1 pound potatoes, peeled
   and diced

1 onion, diced

2 celery stalks, diced

½ cup corn kernels, fresh
   or frozen

½ teaspoon salt

¼ teaspoon freshly ground
   black pepper

¾ pound raw shrimp, peeled and
   deveined

1 pound white fish fillets, cut into
   1-inch pieces

Fresh parsley, for garnish

1. In the slow cooker, combine the water, half-and-half, potatoes, onion, celery, corn, salt, and pepper. Stir to mix well.

2. Cook on low for 3 to 4 hours.

3. Add the shrimp and fish and cook for an additional 15 to 20 minutes.

4. Garnish with parsley just before serving.

INGREDIENT TIP: You can use whatever mild white fish you like; try tilapia, halibut, or haddock. You can even use a darker fish, like salmon. Fresh is best, but you can substitute frozen and thawed seafood.

PER SERVING Calories: 351; Total Fat: 2g; Saturated Fat: 0g; Cholesterol: 125mg; Sodium: 463mg; Potassium: 526mg; Carbs: 35g; Fiber: 4g; Protein: 44g

Chicken and White Bean Soup

SERVES 4 • **PREP TIME:** 10 MINUTES, PLUS OVERNIGHT TO SOAK THE BEANS
COOK TIME: 5 TO 7 HOURS ON LOW

LOW SODIUM

ALLERGY-FRIENDLY • GLUTEN-FREE

This recipe is high in protein, since it has both chicken and beans, making it a satisfying meal on a chilly afternoon. It also happens to be really simple. With the meat, veggies, beans, and seasonings, you don't need much added salt, if any at all.

1½ pounds chicken breasts, boneless and skinless, cut into 1-inch chunks

1 pound white beans, soaked overnight

1 (15-ounce) can no-salt-added diced tomatoes

4 cups low-sodium chicken

3 carrots, diced

2 celery stalks, diced

1 large onion, diced

3 garlic cloves, minced

2 dried bay leaves

1 teaspoon dried basil

1 teaspoon dried oregano

1 teaspoon dried thyme

Salt

Freshly ground black pepper

1. In the slow cooker, combine the chicken, beans, tomatoes and their juices, broth, carrots, celery, onion, garlic, bay leaves, basil, oregano, and thyme, and season lightly with salt and pepper. Stir to mix well.

2. Cook on low for 5 to 7 hours.

3. Remove the bay leaves and serve.

INGREDIENT TIP: Use whatever white beans you have in the pantry: cannellini, great northern, or navy. In a pinch, this can even be Chicken and Pink Bean Soup.

PER SERVING Calories: 632; Total Fat: 4g; Saturated Fat: 0g; Cholesterol: 98mg; Sodium: 285mg; Potassium: 2,529mg; Carbs: 83g; Fiber: 11g; Protein: 70g

Chicken Tortilla Soup

SERVES 4 • PREP TIME: 5 MINUTES, PLUS OVERNIGHT TO SOAK THE BEANS
COOK TIME: 5 TO 7 HOURS ON LOW

LOW SODIUM

ALLERGY-FRIENDLY

A Latin favorite, chicken tortilla soup isn't necessarily thought of as healthy. But if you look at the ingredients list, you'll see that it is. Make it in the slow cooker, and it's super easy, too. Top this soup with tortilla strips, sour cream, avocado, and/or grated cheese.

5 cups low-sodium chicken broth

1 pound boneless, skinless chicken breasts

1 pound dry black beans, soaked overnight

1 pound corn kernels, fresh or frozen

1 (15-ounce) can no-salt-added diced tomatoes

1 onion, diced

3 garlic cloves, minced

1 tablespoon chili powder

2 teaspoons ground cumin

1 teaspoon paprika

½ teaspoon ground coriander

Juice of 1 lime

Salt

Freshly ground black pepper

¼ cup chopped fresh cilantro

1. In the slow cooker, combine the broth, chicken breasts, beans, corn, tomatoes and their juices, onion, garlic, chili powder, cumin, paprika, coriander, and lime juice, and season lightly with salt and pepper.

2. Cook on low for 5 to 7 hours.

3. Transfer the chicken to a platter, shred it with two forks, and return it to the slow cooker.

4. Sprinkle with cilantro before serving.

COOKING TIP: It's okay to use canned beans or corn, but find a no-salt-added or low-sodium version and remember to drain and rinse them first.

PER SERVING Calories: 720; Total Fat: 24g; Saturated Fat: 1g; Cholesterol: 96mg; Sodium: 310mg; Potassium: 2,050mg; Carbs: 106g; Fiber: 21g; Protein: 62g

Turkey and Wild Rice Soup

SERVES 6 • **PREP TIME:** 10 MINUTES • **COOK TIME:** 6 TO 8 HOURS ON LOW

LOW SODIUM

ALLERGY-FRIENDLY • GLUTEN-FREE • LOW-CARB

This easy soup cooks the rice with the rest of the ingredients directly in the slow cooker. If you have leftover cooked turkey lying around, you can use it in place of the raw turkey in this recipe without having to make any modifications to the cook time.

6 cups low-sodium chicken broth or water

¾ pound boneless, skinless turkey, chopped

1 cup uncooked wild rice

1 small onion, chopped

3 celery stalks, diced

2 carrots, sliced

4 ounces mushrooms, sliced

¾ teaspoon salt

½ teaspoon freshly ground black pepper

1 dried bay leaf

1 teaspoon extra-virgin olive oil

Fresh rosemary, for garnish (optional)

1. In the slow cooker, combine the broth, turkey, rice, onion, celery, carrots, mushrooms, salt, pepper, bay leaf, and olive oil. Stir to mix well.

2. Cook on low for 6 to 8 hours.

3. Remove the bay leaf before serving, and garnish with the rosemary (if using).

VARIATION: To make this soup creamier, mix together ¼ cup of water and 2 teaspoons of arrowroot or potato starch. When the soup is done, stir this slurry into the slow cooker and heat for 5 to 15 minutes more, or until thickened.

PER SERVING Calories: 210; Total Fat: 2g; Saturated Fat: 0g; Cholesterol: 39mg; Sodium: 419mg; Potassium: 453mg; Carbs: 25g; Fiber: 3g; Protein: 20g

Italian Wedding Soup

SERVES 4 • **PREP TIME:** 15 MINUTES • **COOK TIME:** 5 HOURS 15 MINUTES
TO 7 HOURS 15 MINUTES ON LOW

LOW SODIUM

LOW-CARB

Italian wedding soup actually doesn't have anything to do with weddings. The term "wedding soup" comes from the Italian phrase "minestra maritata," which is a reference to the flavor produced by the "marriage" of greens and broth. You can use any kind of pasta; it doesn't have to be orzo. Use another ¼ cup of grated Parmesan cheese to top this soup off perfectly.

For the meatballs

1 pound lean ground beef

1 garlic clove, minced

1 large egg

¼ cup finely chopped onion

¼ cup freshly grated
Parmesan cheese

1 teaspoon dried parsley

1 teaspoon dried oregano

½ teaspoon salt

¼ teaspoon freshly ground
black pepper

For the soup

8 cups low-sodium chicken broth

2 carrots, peeled and chopped

1 onion, diced

1 tablespoon dried parsley

1 teaspoon dried oregano

2 garlic cloves, minced

1½ cups uncooked orzo pasta

4 ounces fresh baby spinach

To make the meatballs

In a large bowl, mix to combine the beef, garlic, egg, onion, cheese, parsley, oregano, salt, and pepper. Shape into 1-inch balls.

To make the soup

1. Put the meatballs in the slow cooker, and add the broth, carrots, onion, parsley, oregano, and garlic. Stir gently.

2. Cook on low for 5 to 7 hours.

3. Stir in the pasta and spinach and cook for an additional 15 minutes, or until the pasta is soft, and serve.

COOKING TIP: You can premake a big batch of meatballs and freeze them raw. Then simply drop them into the soup frozen at the start of cooking time.

PER SERVING Calories: 344; Total Fat: 11g; Saturated Fat: 4g; Cholesterol: 116mg; Sodium: 345mg; Potassium: 338mg; Carbs: 26g; Fiber: 3g; Protein: 34g

Pork Pho

LOW SODIUM

Pho (pronounced fuh) is a healthy and flavorful Vietnamese soup made with broth, rice noodles, fresh herbs, and some meat. It's a kind of street food in Vietnam, and it made its way around the world with Vietnamese immigrants. Beef and chicken tend to be the most popular meats, but this version calls for pork. If you don't have tenderloin, you can just cut the bone out of a few pork chops, or try boneless beef ribs or chicken thighs.

1 pound pork tenderloin, cut into thin slices

6 cups low-sodium chicken broth

2 teaspoons low-sodium soy sauce (or tamari if gluten-free)

1 small onion, chopped

⅓ cup peeled and sliced fresh ginger

3 garlic cloves, minced

1 teaspoon ground coriander

½ teaspoon ground cumin

2 teaspoons honey

¼ teaspoon salt

8 ounces rice noodles

1. In the slow cooker, combine the pork, broth, soy sauce, onion, ginger, garlic, coriander, cumin, honey, and salt. Stir to mix well.

2. Cook on low for 4 to 6 hours.

3. Stir in the noodles. Cook for an additional 10 minutes, or until the noodles are tender, and serve.

COOKING TIP: You can add almost anything to a bowl of pho. Try serving it with lime wedges, fresh cilantro, sliced scallions, bean sprouts, fresh sliced bird's-eye or habanero chiles, or sriracha sauce.

PER SERVING Calories: 393; Total Fat: 4g; Saturated Fat: 2g; Cholesterol: 75mg; Sodium: 314mg; Potassium: 59mg; Carbs: 55g; Fiber: 1g; Protein: 29g

Indian Vegetable Stew

SERVES 4 • **PREP TIME:** 10 MINUTES • **COOK TIME:** 3 TO 4 HOURS ON LOW

LOW SODIUM

ALLERGY-FRIENDLY • GLUTEN-FREE • LOW-CHOLESTEROL • VEGAN

While some people might call this a curry, it's technically a spiced stew. Stews and curries have a lot in common, and sometimes they are hard to differentiate. In general, if you can drink the liquid, then it's a stew. Using 4 cups of water gives this dish the consistency of a stew. If the flavor is too strong, reduce the curry powder from 1 tablespoon to 1½ teaspoons.

1 (15-ounce) can chickpeas, drained and rinsed

4 cups water

1 (15-ounce) can no-salt-added diced tomatoes

2 medium sweet potatoes, peeled and diced

1 medium onion, diced

1 bell pepper, seeded and diced

2 garlic cloves, minced

1 tablespoon curry powder

1½ teaspoons ground ginger

½ teaspoon salt

1 teaspoon ground cumin

1 teaspoon ground turmeric

1 teaspoon ground coriander

1 teaspoon red pepper flakes

½ pint cherry tomatoes, halved

½ cup frozen peas

Chopped fresh parsley, for garnish (optional)

1. In the slow cooker, combine the chickpeas, water, tomatoes and their juices, sweet potatoes, onion, bell pepper, garlic, curry powder, ginger, salt, cumin, turmeric, coriander, and red pepper flakes. Stir to mix well.

2. Cook on low for 2½ to 3½ hours.

3. When there are 30 minutes of cooking time left, stir in the cherry tomatoes and peas. Mix well and cook for the remaining 30 minutes.

4. Garnish with parsley (if using) and serve.

VARIATION: For a richer flavor, use low-sodium broth instead of water. You can easily turn this into a soup by adding an additional 2 cups of liquid.

PER SERVING Calories: 267; Total Fat: 3g; Saturated Fat: 0g; Cholesterol: 0mg; Sodium: 356mg; Potassium: 924mg; Carbs: 51g; Fiber: 13g; Protein: 12g

Moroccan Chickpea Stew

SERVES 4 • **PREP TIME:** 10 MINUTES, PLUS OVERNIGHT TO SOAK THE BEANS
COOK TIME: 5 TO 7 HOURS ON LOW

LOW SODIUM

ALLERGY-FRIENDLY

North African cuisine tends to use very aromatic and flavorful combinations of spices, many of which are captured in this recipe. Using chickpeas and vegetables, this hearty stew is the epitome of healthy comfort food.

1 pound boneless, skinless chicken thighs

½ pound dry chickpeas, soaked overnight

5 cups low-sodium chicken broth

1 (15-ounce) can no-salt-added diced tomatoes

1 onion, diced

4 garlic cloves, minced

1 teaspoon ground ginger

1 teaspoon ground cumin

1 teaspoon ground turmeric

1 teaspoon paprika

1 teaspoon red pepper flakes

1 teaspoon ground cinnamon

1 teaspoon ground coriander

1 teaspoon ground nutmeg

1 teaspoon ground cloves

½ teaspoon salt

½ teaspoon freshly ground black pepper

¼ cup chopped fresh cilantro or parsley

1. In the slow cooker, combine the chicken, chickpeas, broth, tomatoes, onion, garlic, ginger, cumin, turmeric, paprika, red pepper flakes, cinnamon, coriander, nutmeg, cloves, salt, and pepper. Stir to mix well.

2. Cook on low for 5 to 7 hours.

3. Top with the cilantro and serve.

COOKING TIP: You can use one 15-ounce can of chickpeas instead of the dried ones. Just drain and rinse them first.

PER SERVING Calories: 431; Total Fat: 28g; Saturated Fat: 2g; Cholesterol: 126mg; Sodium: 329mg; Potassium: 886mg; Carbs: 45g; Fiber: 13g; Protein: 41g

Gumbo

SERVES 8 • **PREP TIME:** 10 MINUTES • **COOK TIME:** 6 HOURS 10 MINUTES
TO 8 HOURS 15 MINUTES ON LOW

LOWER SODIUM

LOW-CARB

Most gumbos require a roux—flour and fat cooked together, which is then used to thicken sauces. To keep things healthy, I've skipped the roux and relied on the okra as a natural thickener. You might be tempted to add broth or water, but they aren't needed. The natural juices of all the ingredients will create a wonderful, thick gravy.

2 to 3 pounds boneless, skinless chicken thighs

½ pound Breakfast Sausage (page 48)

1 bell pepper, seeded and diced

1 onion, diced

2 celery stalks, finely chopped

4 garlic cloves

2 dried bay leaves

1 cup frozen okra

¾ cup no-salt-added tomato paste

1 (15-ounce) can no-salt-added diced tomatoes

1 tablespoon plus 1 teaspoon Homemade Cajun Blend (page 8)

½ teaspoon freshly ground black pepper

½ teaspoon ground cayenne pepper

½ teaspoon dried thyme

½ teaspoon dried oregano

1 pound raw shrimp, peeled and deveined

1. In the slow cooker, combine the chicken, sausage, bell pepper, onion, celery, garlic, bay leaves, okra, tomato paste, tomatoes and their juices, Cajun blend, black pepper, cayenne pepper, thyme, and oregano. Stir to mix well.

2. Cook on low for 6 to 8 hours.

3. Gently stir in the shrimp. Cover and cook for about 10 to 15 minutes more, or until the shrimp are pink and cooked through.

4. Remove the bay leaves before serving.

COOKING TIP: Serve this dish over rice, or even cauliflower rice.

PER SERVING Calories: 306; Total Fat: 11g; Saturated Fat: 3g; Cholesterol: 205mg; Sodium: 243mg; Potassium: 585mg; Carbs: 11g; Fiber: 3g; Protein: 41g

Pork Cider Stew

SERVES 6 • **PREP TIME:** 10 MINUTES • **COOK TIME:** 4 TO 6 HOURS ON LOW

LOW SODIUM

ALLERGY-FRIENDLY • LOW-CARB

Cider is often paired with pork when slow cooking because its acidic tang will tenderize the meat, while its fruity undertone adds just the right amount of sweetness. With the addition of potatoes and vegetables, this hearty pork stew will certainly stick to your ribs.

2½ pounds boneless pork shoulder, fat trimmed, cut into 1-inch cubes

1 cup cider

2 cups no-salt-added beef broth

½ pound red or yellow potatoes, chopped

2 carrots, chopped

3 celery stalks, chopped

1 large apple, cored and chopped

1 onion, diced

½ tablespoon Dijon mustard

1 tablespoon apple cider vinegar

1½ teaspoons dried thyme

1 teaspoon dried rosemary

½ teaspoon salt

½ teaspoon freshly ground black pepper

1. In the slow cooker, combine the pork, cider, broth, potatoes, carrots, celery, apple, onion, mustard, vinegar, thyme, rosemary, salt, and pepper. Stir to mix well.

2. Cook on low for 4 to 6 hours, or until both the pork and the potatoes are tender, and serve.

VARIATION: You can use cut-up country pork ribs rather than pork shoulder. Swap out the potatoes for sweet potatoes or even butternut squash.

PER SERVING Calories: 279; Total Fat: 6g; Saturated Fat: 2g; Cholesterol: 108mg; Sodium: 299mg; Potassium: 368mg; Carbs: 21g; Fiber: 3g; Protein: 36g

Peruvian Beef Stew

SERVES 4 • **PREP TIME:** 10 MINUTES • **COOK TIME:** 6 TO 8 HOURS ON LOW

LOW SODIUM

ALLERGY-FRIENDLY • GLUTEN-FREE • LOW-CARB

Latin flavors spice up this hearty and healthy stew. Some variations on this recipe include beans and peas, and you can certainly add a can of beans (drained and rinsed) and/or a cup of frozen peas at the start of cooking.

1½ pounds beef stew meat

3 cups Beef Bone Broth (page 24)

1 onion, diced

1 bell pepper, seeded and diced

½ pound potatoes, diced

3 large carrots, peeled and chopped

2 dried bay leaves

3 garlic cloves, chopped

2 teaspoons ground cumin

½ teaspoon salt

¼ teaspoon freshly ground black pepper

1 bunch cilantro, stemmed and finely chopped

1. In the slow cooker, combine the stew meat, broth, onion, bell pepper, potatoes, carrots, bay leaves, garlic, cumin, salt, and pepper. Stir to mix well.

2. Cook on low for 6 to 8 hours.

3. Remove the bay leaves and garnish with fresh cilantro before serving.

VARIATION: Kick this stew up a couple of notches by adding a spicy element, such as a diced hot pepper or a dash of hot pepper sauce.

PER SERVING Calories: 341; Total Fat: 9g; Saturated Fat: 3g; Cholesterol: 113mg; Sodium: 487mg; Potassium: 534mg; Carbs: 21g; Fiber: 4g; Protein: 42g

STUFFED PEPPERS, PAGE 106

6

Meatless MAINS

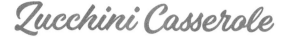

Zucchini Casserole

LOW SODIUM

ALLERGY-FRIENDLY • GLUTEN-FREE • LOW-CARB • LOW-CHOLESTEROL • VEGAN

This light, low-carb, gluten-free zucchini casserole is really easy to throw together, and it's vegan if you leave out the cheese. It's a good recipe to use to clean out your produce drawer. Got carrots? Add those in. A few florets of broccoli? Toss those in, too. See where I'm going here?

3 zucchini, chopped

3 cups Marinara Sauce (page 30)

1 onion, diced

1 green bell pepper, seeded and diced

2 garlic cloves, minced

2 teaspoons Homemade Italian Blend (page 9)

1 teaspoon salt

1 cup shredded low-fat mozzarella cheese (optional, omit if vegan)

1. In the slow cooker, combine the zucchini, marinara sauce, onion, bell pepper, garlic, Italian blend, and salt. Stir to mix well.

2. Cook on low for 3 to 4 hours.

3. Add the cheese (if using) and cook an additional 10 to 20 minutes, or until the cheese is melted, and serve.

VARIATION: For a creamy spin on this casserole, use Alfredo Sauce (page 31) instead of the Marinara Sauce.

PER SERVING Calories: 83; Total Fat: 1g; Saturated Fat: 1g; Cholesterol: 3mg; Sodium: 448mg; Potassium: 795mg; Carbs: 16g; Fiber: 4g; Protein: 5g

Butternut Squash with Sage and Green Beans

SERVES 4 • PREP TIME: 10 MINUTES • COOK TIME: 3 TO 5 HOURS ON LOW

LOW SODIUM

GLUTEN-FREE • LOW-CHOLESTEROL • VEGETARIAN

While the butternut squash and sage may seem heavy, this dish is anything but. The aroma may be strong and savory, but this is a healthy and light vegetarian dish.

2 pounds butternut squash, peeled, seeded, and diced

2 pounds green beans, trimmed and cut into 1-inch pieces

3 tablespoons chopped fresh sage

1 cup low-sodium vegetable broth

¼ cup grated Parmesan cheese

½ teaspoon salt

¼ teaspoon freshly ground black pepper

1 teaspoon unsalted butter (optional)

Red peppercorns, for garnish (optional)

1. In the slow cooker, combine the squash, beans, sage, broth, cheese, salt, pepper, butter, and peppercorns (if using). Stir to mix well.
2. Cook on low for 3 to 5 hours and serve.

SUBSTITUTION TIP: If you're lactose-intolerant but like the flavor of butter, try replacing it with ghee. Ghee is clarified butter that's lactose-free. Parmesan cheese contains less than 0.5 grams of lactose per ounce and can usually be digested by most people who are lactose-intolerant.

PER SERVING Calories: 204; Total Fat: 2g; Saturated Fat: 1g; Cholesterol: 5mg; Sodium: 396mg; Potassium: 1,290mg; Carbs: 44g; Fiber: 13g; Protein: 9g

Spaghetti Squash Pizza Casserole

SERVES 6 • PREP TIME: 10 MINUTES • **COOK TIME:** 2 TO 4 HOURS ON LOW,
PLUS 45 MINUTES TO ROAST

LOW SODIUM

GLUTEN-FREE • LOW-CARB • LOW-CHOLESTEROL • VEGETARIAN

This is a fun recipe to make because there are no limits when it comes to what vegetables you can add. Load those veggies in this dish. Mushrooms, olives, kale, spinach, and peppers all make great additions to this recipe. Whatever you would add to a pizza, add it here. Right in your slow cooker, you get to design your favorite low-carb, vegetarian pizza. If you have a pizza seasoning mix you like, feel free to swap that for the Italian Blend.

1 medium spaghetti squash
(about 2 pounds)

3 cups Marinara Sauce (page 30)

1½ tablespoons Homemade
Italian Blend (page 9)

2 garlic cloves, minced

1 cup any diced vegetables

½ teaspoon salt

¼ cup chopped fresh basil

2 cups shredded low-fat
mozzarella cheese

1. Preheat the oven to 400°F.
2. Halve the squash, and scrape out the seeds. Lay the squash halves cut-side down on a roasting pan and cook for 30 to 45 minutes, until tender when pierced with a fork. Cool slightly.
3. Shred the spaghetti squash with a fork and transfer to a large bowl. Toss with the marinara sauce, Italian blend, and garlic until well combined.
4. Add the squash mixture, vegetables, salt, and basil to the slow cooker. Stir to mix well, and top with the cheese.
5. Cook on low for 2 to 4 hours and serve.

COOKING TIP: Spaghetti squash releases liquid when it cooks, so don't be surprised if the finished product is a little wet.

PER SERVING Calories: 106; Total Fat: 1g; Saturated Fat: 0g; Cholesterol: 1mg; Sodium: 318mg; Potassium: 665mg; Carbs: 21g; Fiber: 2g; Protein: 6g

Spaghetti Squash, Kale, and Mushroom Casserole

SERVES 6 • **PREP TIME:** 10 MINUTES • **COOK TIME:** 4 TO 6 HOURS ON LOW, PLUS 45 MINUTES TO ROAST

LOW SODIUM

GLUTEN-FREE • LOW-CARB • LOW-CHOLESTEROL • VEGETARIAN

Spaghetti squash is a healthy, low-carb alternative to pasta. It's a great replacement in casseroles as well, because it's light yet filling. For an even heartier meal, substitute 8 ounces of cooked regular, gluten-free, or whole-wheat pasta in place of the spaghetti squash.

1 medium spaghetti squash (about 2 pounds)

Nonstick cooking spray

3 cups Marinara Sauce (page 30) or Alfredo Sauce (page 31)

½ teaspoon salt

¼ teaspoon freshly ground black pepper

2 garlic cloves, minced

8 ounces mushrooms, sliced

½ pound kale, chopped

4 cups low-fat mozzarella cheese

1. Preheat the oven to 400°F.
2. Halve the squash and scrape out the seeds. Lay the squash halves cut-side down on a roasting pan and cook for 30 to 45 minutes, until tender when pierced with a fork. Cool slightly.
3. Spray the slow cooker generously with nonstick cooking spray.
4. Shred the spaghetti squash with a fork, and transfer to a large bowl along with the marinara sauce, salt, pepper, and garlic.
5. Gently stir in the mushrooms and kale. Add the entire mixture to the slow cooker. Top with the cheese, and season lightly with salt and pepper.
6. Cook on low for 4 to 6 hours and serve.

INGREDIENT TIP: Spaghetti squash contains lots of potassium, which is so important for balancing the sodium in your diet, as well as vitamin A, folic acid, and beta carotene.

PER SERVING Calories: 169; Total Fat: 4g; Saturated Fat: 2g; Cholesterol: 13mg; Sodium: 373mg; Potassium: 924mg; Carbs: 26g; Fiber: 3g; Protein: 11g

Shepherd's Pie with Mashed Cauliflower

SERVES 6 • **PREP TIME:** 15 MINUTES • **COOK TIME:** 4 HOURS 30 MINUTES TO 6 HOURS 30 MINUTES ON LOW

LOW SODIUM

LOW-CARB • LOW-CHOLESTEROL • VEGETARIAN

Mushrooms replace meat in this vegetarian, low-carb shepherd's pie. Portobello mushrooms are a particularly good choice because of their meaty texture. If you prefer the traditional potato topping, use about 2 pounds of potatoes instead of the head of cauliflower, and just follow the recipe as written.

For the filling

Nonstick cooking spray

1½ pounds mushrooms, sliced

1 tablespoon unsalted butter (or coconut oil if vegan)

1 medium onion, diced

2 garlic cloves, minced

½ cup peas, fresh or frozen

½ cup carrots, peeled and finely chopped

⅓ cup low-sodium vegetable broth

2 tablespoons no-salt-added tomato paste

2 tablespoons almond flour (optional)

¾ teaspoon salt

1 teaspoon dried thyme

½ teaspoon freshly ground black pepper

To make the filling

1. Spray the slow cooker generously with nonstick cooking spray.

2. In the slow cooker, combine the mushrooms, butter, onion, garlic, peas, carrots, broth, tomato paste, almond flour (if using), salt, thyme, and pepper. Stir to mix well.

3. Cook on low for 4 to 6 hours.

For the mashed cauliflower

1 pound cauliflower florets (about 1 small head)

1 teaspoon unsalted butter (or extra-virgin olive oil if vegan)

2 to 3 tablespoons low-fat milk, plus more if needed (or almond milk if vegan)

¼ teaspoon salt

¼ teaspoon freshly ground black pepper

To make the mashed cauliflower

1. Meanwhile, in a microwave-safe covered dish filled with about a half inch of water or in a steamer pot on the stove, steam the cauliflower until tender.

2. In a food processor, combine the cauliflower, butter, milk, salt, and pepper. Pulse until smooth, adding more milk if necessary. Alternatively, mash with a handheld potato masher.

3. Pour the mashed cauliflower on top of the cooked pie filling in the slow cooker. Cook for an additional 30 minutes and serve.

COOKING TIP: This recipe may look like a lot of work, but it's really not. You can make the cauliflower mash while the filling is cooking, or even make it the day before.

PER SERVING Calories: 96; Total Fat: 3g; Saturated Fat: 1g; Cholesterol: 5mg; Sodium: 458mg; Potassium: 721mg; Carbs: 14g; Fiber: 4g; Protein: 6g

Buffalo Cauliflower and Chickpeas

SERVES 4 • **PREP TIME:** 10 MINUTES • **COOK TIME:** 2 TO 4 HOURS ON LOW

LOW SODIUM

LOW-CHOLESTEROL • VEGETARIAN

You should be able to easily find a low-sodium version of your favorite brand of hot sauce in your local grocery. A little bit of buffalo sauce goes a long way, though. If it looks like there's not enough sauce when the food first starts to cook, don't worry—there is.

2 tablespoons low-sodium hot sauce

1 head cauliflower (about 4 cups), chopped

1 (15-ounce) can chickpeas, drained and rinsed

¾ cup low-fat milk (or soy or almond milk if vegan)

3 teaspoons unsalted butter (or coconut oil if vegan)

½ cup water

¼ cup all-purpose flour

2 teaspoons garlic powder

1 teaspoon ground cumin

1 teaspoon paprika

1. In the slow cooker, combine the hot sauce, cauliflower, chickpeas, milk, butter, water, flour, garlic powder, cumin, and paprika. Stir to mix well.

2. Cook on low for 2 to 4 hours and serve.

SUBSTITUTION TIP: Substitute the same amount of gluten-free flour or even almond flour, depending on your dietary needs.

PER SERVING Calories: 272; Total Fat: 7g; Saturated Fat: 4g; Cholesterol: 2mg; Sodium: 434mg; Potassium: 987mg; Carbs: 43g; Fiber: 12g; Protein: 14g

Barbecue Chickpeas

SERVES 6 TO 8 • **PREP TIME:** 10 MINUTES, PLUS OVERNIGHT TO SOAK THE CHICKPEAS
COOK TIME: 6 TO 8 HOURS ON LOW

LOW SODIUM

ALLERGY-FRIENDLY • GLUTEN-FREE • LOW-CHOLESTEROL • VEGETARIAN

Chickpeas are used a lot in slow cooking, and not just for their nutritional value. They're also quite sturdy, so they tend to maintain their shape during the low slow cooking. Slow cooking these chickpeas in homemade barbecue sauce means the flavor really gets into the beans rather than simply clinging to the surface.

1 pound dry chickpeas, soaked overnight

2 cups Ketchup (page 25)

1 cup water

1 small onion, diced

2 celery stalks, diced

¼ cup extra-virgin olive oil

¼ cup freshly squeezed lemon juice

¼ cup apple cider vinegar

¼ cup maple syrup

1 tablespoon powdered mustard

1½ teaspoons gluten-free Worcestershire sauce

¾ teaspoon salt

½ teaspoon freshly ground black pepper

1. In the slow cooker, combine the chickpeas, ketchup, water, onion, celery, olive oil, lemon juice, vinegar, maple syrup, mustard, Worcestershire sauce, salt, and pepper. Stir to mix well.

2. Cook on low for 6 to 8 hours and serve.

COOKING TIP: Top these chickpeas with a homemade coleslaw before serving for a complete meal with veggies.

PER SERVING Calories: 440; Total Fat: 13g; Saturated Fat: 2g; Cholesterol: 0mg; Sodium: 485mg; Potassium: 1,112mg; Carbs: 68g; Fiber: 16g; Protein: 17g

Mexican Beans and Brown Rice

SERVES 6 • **PREP TIME:** 10 MINUTES, PLUS OVERNIGHT TO SOAK THE BEANS
COOK TIME: 4 TO 6 HOURS ON LOW

LOW SODIUM

ALLERGY-FRIENDLY • GLUTEN-FREE • LOW-CHOLESTEROL • VEGAN

Mexican flavors like cumin and chili powder jazz up what would otherwise be a simple dish of beans and rice. Using dry beans and brown rice, this recipe is packed with fiber. Don't like black beans? Substitute pinto beans. Topping options include low-fat sour cream, low-fat cheese, avocado, and shredded greens.

1 pound dry black beans, soaked overnight

1 onion, sliced

1 bell pepper, seeded and diced

2 celery stalks, diced

1 garlic clove, minced

1 teaspoon ground cumin

1 teaspoon chili powder

1 teaspoon paprika

1 teaspoon salt

½ teaspoon freshly ground black pepper

½ teaspoon dried thyme

1 dried bay leaf

6 cups water

4 cups cooked brown rice, warm or room temperature

1. In the slow cooker, combine the beans, onion, bell pepper, celery, garlic, cumin, chili powder, paprika, salt, pepper, thyme, bay leaf, and water. Stir to mix well.
2. Cook on low for 4 to 6 hours, and remove the bay leaf.
3. Stir the brown rice into the slow cooker, stirring gently until well combined, and serve.

COOKING TIP: Brown rice takes a while to cook, but it actually freezes very well. Cook up a big batch and freeze it in 1-cup bags. Thaw overnight in the fridge, and toss it into any recipe that calls for cooked rice.

PER SERVING Calories: 380; Total Fat: 2g; Saturated Fat: 0g; Cholesterol: 0mg; Sodium: 402mg; Potassium: 1,323mg; Carbs: 73g; Fiber: 13g; Protein: 19g

Stuffed Acorn Squash

SERVES 2 • **PREP TIME:** 10 MINUTES • **COOK TIME:** 6 TO 8 HOURS ON LOW

LOWEST SODIUM

GLUTEN-FREE • LOW-CHOLESTEROL • VEGETARIAN

This sweet and savory squash recipe for two might be a single or double serving, depending on the size of your squash. This is a recipe that uses autumn produce, so feel free to mix things up with the autumn fruits; rather than an apple, try a pear.

1 cup cooked brown rice

1 small apple, cored and diced

2 tablespoons dried cranberries

2 tablespoons chopped nuts (pecans, almonds, walnuts)

2 teaspoons unsalted butter (or extra-virgin olive oil if vegan), divided

1 acorn squash, halved and seeded

2 tablespoons honey (or maple syrup if vegan)

1 teaspoon ground cinnamon

¼ teaspoon ground nutmeg

1. In a large bowl, mix together the rice, apple, cranberries, and nuts.

2. Put 1 teaspoon of butter in each squash half, and fill the halves with the rice mixture.

3. Pour 1 cup of water into the bottom of the slow cooker. Place the stuffed squash in the bottom of the slow cooker, stuffed-side up.

4. In a small bowl, mix together the honey, cinnamon, and nutmeg. Sprinkle over the squash and filling.

5. Cook on low for 6 to 8 hours, or until the squash is tender, and serve.

VARIATION: For a low-carb, grain-free version, use an equal amount of grated cauliflower (cauliflower rice) instead of the brown rice.

PER SERVING Calories: 382; Total Fat: 10g; Saturated Fat: 1g; Cholesterol: 0mg; Sodium: 66mg; Potassium: 997mg; Carbs: 75g; Fiber: 8g; Protein: 5g

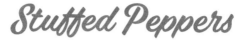

Stuffed Peppers

SERVES 2 • **PREP TIME:** 10 MINUTES • **COOK TIME:** 4 HOURS 10 MINUTES
TO 6 HOURS 15 MINUTES ON LOW

LOW SODIUM

GLUTEN-FREE • LOW-CARB • LOW-CHOLESTEROL • VEGETARIAN

Stuffed peppers are a versatile slow cooker meal. They can be made with so many different flavor profiles. This version has an Italian theme using marinara sauce and Italian seasonings. If you have fresh herbs, toss those in on top.

For the filling

½ cup cooked quinoa

1 tablespoon grated
    Parmesan cheese

½ cup Marinara Sauce (page 30)

1 garlic clove, minced

1 tablespoon dried oregano

1½ teaspoons dried basil

¼ teaspoon salt

¼ teaspoon freshly ground
    black pepper

For the bell peppers

Nonstick cooking spray

2 bell peppers

¼ cup sliced fresh
    mozzarella cheese

To make the filling

In a large bowl, mix together the quinoa, Parmesan cheese, marinara sauce, garlic, oregano, basil, salt, and pepper.

To make the bell peppers

1. Spray the slow cooker generously with nonstick cooking spray.

2. To prepare the bell peppers, cut a circle in the top of each pepper around the stem and remove the stem. Use a spoon to carefully remove the pith and seeds. You can turn the pepper over to shake out some of the loose seeds. Spoon the filling into each bell pepper cavity.

3. Place the stuffed bell peppers in the slow cooker. Cook on low for 4 to 6 hours.

4. Top the peppers with the mozzarella, cover, and cook for an additional 10 to 15 minutes, or until the cheese has melted, and serve.

SUBSTITUTION TIP: Dairy-free or vegan? Omit the cheese. You can also substitute brown rice or even cauliflower rice (a low-carb choice) for the quinoa.

PER SERVING Calories: 187; Total Fat: 6g; Saturated Fat: 4g; Cholesterol: 22mg; Sodium: 345mg; Potassium: 360mg; Carbs: 15g; Fiber: 4g; Protein: 11g

Mushroom Risotto

SERVES 6 • **PREP TIME:** 10 MINUTES • **COOK TIME:** 5 TO 7 HOURS ON LOW

LOW SODIUM

ALLERGY-FRIENDLY • GLUTEN-FREE • LOW-CHOLESTEROL • VEGAN

This dish is for mushroom lovers. Pile them on, and mix it up with all the types of mushrooms you can find. Since the rice is cooked low and slow, this risotto will be a lot softer than the stove top version. It's also different from a traditional risotto in that it's not loaded with butter and cheese. In this healthier version, I've left out the butter entirely, and the cheese is optional.

1¾ cups uncooked rice

4 cups low-sodium vegetable broth

8 ounces mushrooms, diced

2 tablespoons extra-virgin olive oil

1 small onion, chopped

2 garlic cloves, minced

1 teaspoon salt

¼ teaspoon freshly ground black pepper

¼ cup shredded low-fat Asiago or Parmesan cheese (optional, omit if vegan)

1. In the slow cooker, combine the rice, broth, mushrooms, olive oil, onion, garlic, salt, and pepper. Stir to mix well.
2. Cook on low for 5 to 7 hours.
3. Add the cheese, stir, and cook until the cheese is melted, about 10 minutes more, and serve.

VARIATION: Which cheese works best with this will depend on the flavor profile of the mushrooms. Pair Parmigiano-Reggiano or even Gruyère with heartier mushrooms; mozzarella, Parmesan, or Asiago with more delicate flavors.

PER SERVING Calories: 261; Total Fat: 5g; Saturated Fat: 1g; Cholesterol: 0mg; Sodium: 440mg; Potassium: 205mg; Carbs: 47g; Fiber: 1g; Protein: 7g

Pasta Primavera

SERVES 6 • **PREP TIME:** 10 MINUTES • **COOK TIME:** 4 TO 6 HOURS ON LOW

LOW SODIUM

LOW-CHOLESTEROL • VEGETARIAN

Most people don't think of this classic pasta dish as a slow cooker recipe, but it's a great one to dump all the ingredients in and let it cook. You can use your preferred pasta shape and grain. The pasta goes in uncooked to make this recipe not only healthy but super easy.

Nonstick cooking spray

8 ounces uncooked pasta

5 cups Marinara Sauce (page 30)

2 cups broccoli florets

½ cup carrots, peeled and diced

1 bell pepper, seeded and diced

1 small onion, diced

1 zucchini, chopped

1 yellow squash, chopped

½ cup cherry tomatoes, halved

½ cup frozen peas

1½ teaspoons extra-virgin
   olive oil

2 teaspoons Homemade
   Italian Blend (page 9)

2 garlic cloves, minced

½ teaspoon salt

¼ cup grated Parmesan cheese

¼ cup chopped fresh parsley

1. Spray the slow cooker generously with nonstick cooking spray.

2. In the slow cooker, combine the pasta, marinara sauce, broccoli, carrots, bell pepper, onion, zucchini, squash, tomatoes, peas, olive oil, Italian blend, garlic, salt, and cheese. Stir to mix well.

3. Cover and cook on low for 4 to 6 hours.

4. Garnish with the fresh parsley and serve.

INGREDIENT TIP: With some recipes you can swap in frozen vegetables, but this isn't one of them. Pasta Primavera calls for fresh vegetables.

PER SERVING Calories: 295; Total Fat: 4g; Saturated Fat: 1g; Cholesterol: 3mg; Sodium: 320mg; Potassium: 2,370mg; Carbs: 56g; Fiber: 10g; Protein: 13g

Pesto and Cheese–Stuffed Shells

SERVES 4 • **PREP TIME:** 15 MINUTES • **COOK TIME:** 3 TO 4 HOURS ON LOW

LOW SODIUM

VEGETARIAN

While this recipe seems fancy, you can put it together in just a few minutes. There's no need to boil the manicotti shells; they cook in the slow cooker along with all the other ingredients. But be careful because the shells will dry out if they're overcooked. If that happens, try adding more sauce to the slow cooker.

For the stuffing

1 cup shredded low-fat mozzarella cheese

½ cup low-sodium basil pesto, homemade or store-bought

1 cup low-fat cottage cheese

2 tablespoons Homemade Italian Blend (page 9)

For the shells

8 ounces uncooked manicotti shells

7 cups Marinara Sauce (page 30), divided

1 cup shredded low-fat mozzarella cheese

To make the stuffing

1. In a large bowl, mix 1 cup of the mozzarella cheese together with the pesto, cottage cheese, and Italian blend.
2. Transfer the mixture to a large resealable plastic bag and seal it. Cut a little triangle off a bottom corner of the plastic bag.

To make the shells

1. Squeeze the cheese mixture into each of the manicotti shells until they're all stuffed.
2. Pour 3½ cups of marinara sauce into the bottom of the slow cooker. Arrange the stuffed manicotti shells on top. Pour the remaining 3½ cups of sauce on top of the shells so all the shells are covered.
3. Cook on low for 2½ to 3½ hours.
4. Sprinkle the mozzarella cheese on top, cook for 30 minutes more, and serve.

VARIATION: Add ½ cup of your favorite chopped vegetables, such as bell pepper, onion, mushrooms, or zucchini, to the cheese mixture.

PER SERVING Calories: 698; Total Fat: 26g; Saturated Fat: 6g; Cholesterol: 27mg; Sodium: 348mg; Potassium: 2,121mg; Carbs: 82g; Fiber: 12g; Protein: 33g

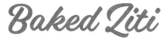

Baked Ziti

SERVES 6 • **PREP TIME:** 10 MINUTES • **COOK TIME:** 4 HOURS 15 MINUTES
TO 6 HOURS 30 MINUTES ON LOW

LOW SODIUM

LOW-CHOLESTEROL • VEGETARIAN

No boiling required! The pasta goes in uncooked, which makes this traditional and impressive baked pasta casserole even easier. Grab your favorite vegetables for this; you can use the mushrooms and zucchini listed here, or add spinach, kale, or whatever is in season today.

1 (28-ounce) can no-salt-added
   diced tomatoes

2½ cups Marinara Sauce
   (page 30)

2½ cups low-sodium
   vegetable broth

½ pound mushrooms, sliced

½ pound zucchini, sliced

1 onion, chopped

2 garlic cloves, minced

½ teaspoon salt

1 teaspoon dried basil

1 teaspoon dried parsley

1 pound uncooked ziti

1 cup shredded low-fat
   mozzarella cheese

1. In the slow cooker, combine the tomatoes, marinara sauce, broth, mushrooms, zucchini, onion, garlic, salt, basil, and parsley. Stir to mix well.

2. Cook on low for 4 to 6 hours.

3. Stir in the uncooked pasta, and top with the mozzarella cheese. Cook for an additional 15 to 30 minutes, or until the pasta is tender and the cheese is melted, and serve.

COOKING TIP: Before you add the pasta to the slow cooker, run it under some water in a strainer. Slightly wet, uncooked noodles will be less likely to stick together.

PER SERVING Calories: 373; Total Fat: 3g; Saturated Fat: 1g; Cholesterol: 3mg; Sodium: 342mg; Potassium: 965mg; Carbs: 75g; Fiber: 8g; Protein: 16g

Sweet and Spicy Peanut Pasta

SERVES 4 • **PREP TIME:** 10 MINUTES • **COOK TIME:** 3 HOURS 10 MINUTES
TO 5 HOURS 10 MINUTES ON LOW

LOW SODIUM

LOW-CHOLESTEROL • VEGETARIAN

If you have a peanut allergy, sorry, this recipe is not for you. But if you don't, and you like pasta smothered in an unusual, thick, sweet, and spicy sauce, then here you go. This is kind of like the peanut-sesame noodles you get at Asian restaurants.

Nonstick cooking spray

¾ cup honey

2 tablespoons sriracha sauce

1½ tablespoons low-sodium soy sauce or tamari

2 garlic cloves, minced

2 teaspoons dried basil

1 small onion, diced

2 carrots, julienned

1 bell pepper, seeded and diced

2 celery stalks, diced

2 cups peanuts

1 pound uncooked spaghetti

1. Spray the slow cooker generously with nonstick cooking spray.
2. In the base of the slow cooker, whisk together the honey, sriracha, soy sauce, garlic, and basil until well blended.
3. Add the onion, carrots, bell pepper, and celery, and stir to mix well.
4. Cook on low for 3 to 5 hours.
5. Stir in the peanuts.
6. While the peanuts are warming in the slow cooker, cook the pasta on the stove top according to package instructions. Drain well.
7. Serve the sweet and spicy peanut sauce on top of the cooked spaghetti.

SUBSTITUTION TIP: For a gluten-free option, this dish is great with rice noodles, and it ends up being a bit like pad Thai. To go vegan, substitute maple or agave syrup for the honey.

PER SERVING Calories: 823; Total Fat: 38g; Saturated Fat: 5g; Cholesterol: 0mg; Sodium: 492mg; Potassium: 756mg; Carbs: 109g; Fiber: 12g; Protein: 27g

Red Potato and Bell Pepper Casserole

SERVES 4 • **PREP TIME:** 10 MINUTES • **COOK TIME:** 3 HOURS 30 MINUTES
TO 5 HOURS 30 MINUTES ON LOW

LOW SODIUM

ALLERGY-FRIENDLY • GLUTEN-FREE • LOW-CHOLESTEROL • VEGETARIAN

This hearty recipe has the three components of a good casserole: vegetables, a starch, and a cheese topping. It's good enough to impress your vegetarian dinner guests, yet simple enough to serve as a last-minute throw-together meal.

2½ pounds red potatoes, sliced

4 bell peppers, seeded and diced

2 garlic cloves, minced

1 teaspoon paprika

½ teaspoon salt

½ teaspoon dried oregano

½ teaspoon ground coriander

¼ teaspoon freshly ground
black pepper

¾ cup low-sodium
vegetable broth

2 cups shredded low-fat
Cheddar cheese

1. In the slow cooker, combine the potatoes, bell peppers, garlic, paprika, salt, oregano, coriander, and pepper. Pour the broth over the top.

2. Cook on low for 3 to 5 hours, or until the potatoes are tender.

3. Add the cheese and cook for an additional 30 minutes, or until melted, and serve.

SUBSTITUTION TIP: To make this vegan, use a vegan cheese substitute or full-fat coconut milk or coconut cream. Coconut will give it a different flavor profile, though.

PER SERVING Calories: 256; Total Fat: 4g; Saturated Fat: 2g; Cholesterol: 8mg; Sodium: 409mg; Potassium: 1,412mg; Carbs: 50g; Fiber: 6g; Protein: 10g

Sweet Potato Casserole

SERVES 6 • **PREP TIME:** 10 MINUTES • **COOK TIME:** 2 TO 4 HOURS ON LOW

LOW SODIUM

GLUTEN-FREE • LOW-CHOLESTEROL • VEGETARIAN

Sweet and savory sweet potato casserole is usually served around the winter holidays, but it's really a year-round dish. You can change this recipe to meet your specific dietary needs. For example, if you have a dairy allergy, use ghee instead of butter. To add more flavor, use a low-sodium broth instead of the water. You can even use fat-free half-and-half or coconut cream instead of water for a creamier casserole. Serve this casserole with a vegetable side dish—a simple salad will do—for a complete meal.

4 pounds sweet potatoes, peeled and chopped

1 cup water

¼ cup honey or maple syrup

2 teaspoons ground cinnamon

¼ teaspoon ground nutmeg

½ teaspoon salt

1 tablespoon unsalted butter

½ cup coarsely chopped pecans or walnuts, lightly toasted

1. In the slow cooker, combine the potatoes, water, honey, cinnamon, nutmeg, salt, and butter. Stir to mix well.
2. Cook on low for 2 to 4 hours, or until the potatoes are soft.
3. Using an immersion blender, potato masher, or the back of a large spoon, mash the sweet potatoes until they reach your desired consistency.
4. Top with the chopped nuts and serve.

COOKING TIP: You can quickly toast nuts in the microwave. Spread the nuts in a single layer in a flat, microwave-safe dish, drizzle ½ teaspoon extra-virgin olive oil on top, and microwave on high for 1 minute. Toss the nuts gently, and microwave for an additional minute. Repeat until the nuts are toasted to your liking.

PER SERVING Calories: 383; Total Fat: 8g; Saturated Fat: 2g; Cholesterol: 4mg; Sodium: 361mg; Potassium: 1,077mg; Carbs: 75g; Fiber: 10g; Protein: 6g

Barbecue Pulled Jackfruit

SERVES 8 • **PREP TIME:** 10 MINUTES • **COOK TIME:** 6 TO 8 HOURS ON LOW

LOW SODIUM

ALLERGY-FRIENDLY • GLUTEN-FREE • LOW-CHOLESTEROL • VEGETARIAN

Jackfruit is a tropical fruit that is not just rich in fiber but also a good source of magnesium, iron, and potassium. While the flavor can be fruity, the texture is that of a shredded meat when cooked. You'll find it in Asian groceries and health food stores. This pulled vegan pork looks and tastes so much like shredded pork, it would fool even the biggest meat eater.

4 (20-ounce) cans jackfruit, drained and rinsed

2 cups Ketchup (page 25)

1 cup water

1 small onion, diced

2 celery stalks, diced

¼ cup extra-virgin olive oil

¼ cup freshly squeezed lemon juice

¼ cup apple cider vinegar

¼ cup maple syrup

1 tablespoon powdered mustard

1 teaspoon salt

½ teaspoon freshly ground black pepper

1½ teaspoons gluten-free Worcestershire sauce

1. In the slow cooker, combine the jackfruit, ketchup, water, onion, celery, olive oil, lemon juice, vinegar, maple syrup, mustard, salt, pepper, and Worcestershire sauce. Stir to mix well.

2. Cook on low for 6 to 8 hours.

3. Transfer the jackfruit to a plate. Using two forks, twist to pull the jackfruit into shreds. Return it to the cooker and heat through before serving.

COOKING TIP: Serve this barbecue on a bun for a pulled-pork-style sandwich, over greens for a warm salad, or even in a tortilla for tacos.

PER SERVING Calories: 181; Total Fat: 7g; Saturated Fat: 1g; Cholesterol: 0mg; Sodium: 463mg; Potassium: 558mg; Carbs: 31g; Fiber: 3g; Protein: 3g

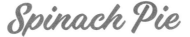

Spinach Pie

SERVES 6 • **PREP TIME:** 10 MINUTES • **COOK TIME:** 1 TO 2 HOURS ON HIGH
AND 6 TO 8 HOURS ON LOW

LOW SODIUM

LOW-CARB • VEGETARIAN

Here is a slow cooker spin on spanakopita, a traditional Greek pastry pie. This pie only uses 1 pie crust on the bottom, so while it might be missing the flaky topping the traditional flavors are still there. Serve this spinach pie hot or at room temperature.

Nonstick cooking spray

1 refrigerated pie crust

1 bunch fresh spinach, chopped

1 tablespoon extra-virgin olive oil

1 small onion, chopped

1 green onion, thinly sliced

½ teaspoon salt

¼ teaspoon freshly ground
    black pepper

¼ teaspoon ground nutmeg

¾ cup crumbled low-fat
    feta cheese

2 cups low-fat ricotta cheese

½ cup grated Parmesan cheese

1 large egg, beaten

1. Spray the slow cooker generously with nonstick cooking spray.

2. Press the pie crust into the bottom of the slow cooker so it comes 1 to 2 inches up the sides.

3. Place a dish towel or 2 paper towels between the slow cooker and the lid. This will absorb the condensation so it won't drip onto the crust while it cooks.

4. Cook on high for 1 to 2 hours.

5. In a large bowl, mix together the spinach, olive oil, onions, salt, pepper, nutmeg, all three cheeses, and the egg. Pour the mixture on top of the pie crust and spread evenly.

6. Cook on low for 6 to 8 hours and serve.

COOKING TIP: You can substitute 30 ounces of chopped frozen spinach, thawed and squeezed to remove excess water, for the fresh spinach if needed.

PER SERVING Calories: 206; Total Fat: 13g; Saturated Fat: 6g; Cholesterol: 54mg; Sodium: 456mg; Potassium: 451mg; Carbs: 10g; Fiber: 2g; Protein: 15g

Savory Mushroom Quiche

SERVES 4 • **PREP TIME:** 15 MINUTES • **COOK TIME:** 1 TO 2 HOURS ON HIGH AND 6 TO 8 HOURS ON LOW

LOW SODIUM

LOW-CARB • VEGETARIAN

Quiche seems to be on a lot of brunch menus, but it can be served any time of the day. This quiche is savory and hearty; I've tried to be as healthy as possible without compromising flavor. Kale can be used instead of spinach. You can also make your own pie crusts using the flour of your choice, rather than using a refrigerated crust.

1 refrigerated pie crust

4 large eggs

4 ounces mushrooms, sliced

¼ cup chopped fresh spinach

2 tablespoons minced onion

1 cup shredded low-fat mozzarella cheese

½ cup low-fat milk or almond milk

1 garlic clove, minced

½ teaspoon salt

⅛ teaspoon freshly ground black pepper

1. Spray the slow cooker generously with nonstick cooking spray or line with parchment paper, covering the bottom and all the way up the sides.

2. Press the pie crust down in the bottom of the slow cooker and up the sides, overlapping so it's one continuous pie crust.

3. Place a small towel or 2 paper towels in between the slow cooker and the lid. This will catch the condensation so it won't drip onto the crust while it cooks.

4. Cook for 1 to 2 hours on high.

5. In a large bowl, whisk together the eggs, mushrooms, spinach, onion, cheese, milk, garlic, salt, and pepper. Pour the filling into the cooked pie crust in the slow cooker.

6. Cook for an additional 6 to 8 hours on low, or until the eggs in the center of the quiche are set and the edges of the crust are browned.

7. Cool for 10 minutes, then lift out, cut, and serve.

COOKING TIP: While nonstick cooking spray will keep the crust from sticking, use parchment paper if you have it. It will make handling the quiche after it's cooked much easier, because you will be able to lift the quiche out of the slow cooker by the edges of the parchment paper.

PER SERVING Calories: 133; Total Fat: 8g; Saturated Fat: 3g; Cholesterol: 170mg; Sodium: 447mg; Potassium: 217mg; Carbs: 7g; Fiber: 1g; Protein: 10g

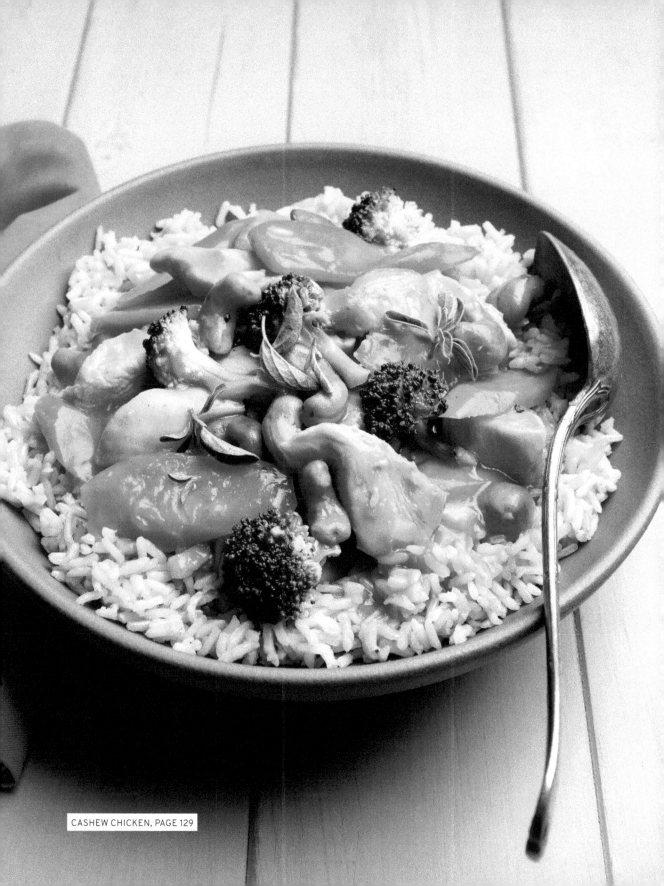

CASHEW CHICKEN, PAGE 129

Chicken and Turkey MAINS

Barbecue Chicken and Onions

SERVES 4 • **PREP TIME:** 5 MINUTES • **COOK TIME:** 4 TO 6 HOURS ON LOW

LOW SODIUM

ALLERGY-FRIENDLY • GLUTEN-FREE • LOW-CARB

Including the homemade barbecue sauce, there are only three ingredients in this recipe. Yet it cooks up a versatile meat that can be used in many different ways. Try pairing it with corn on the cob, or serving it up on a bun with some cole slaw on the side.

1½ pounds boneless, skinless chicken breasts

1 large onion, sliced

1½ cups Barbecue Sauce (page 27)

1. In the slow cooker, combine the chicken, onion, and barbecue sauce. Stir to mix well.
2. Cook on low for 4 to 6 hours and serve.

VARIATION: In the mood for pulled chicken? Remove the cooked chicken, shred it with two forks, and return it to the slow cooker for a few minutes, just to warm it through.

PER SERVING Calories: 262; Total Fat: 2g; Saturated Fat: 1g; Cholesterol: 100mg; Sodium: 411mg; Potassium: 843mg; Carbs: 19g; Fiber: 1g; Protein: 42g

Lemon-Thyme Chicken

SERVES 4 • **PREP TIME:** 5 MINUTES • **COOK TIME:** 5 TO 7 HOURS ON LOW

LOW SODIUM

ALLERGY-FRIENDLY • LOW-CARB

Make this lemon-thyme chicken a one-pot meal by adding a handful of chopped potatoes or sweet potatoes and a handful of chopped vegetables such as green beans. You can add these into the cooker right at the start of cooking, along with the rest of the ingredients.

1 small onion, sliced

2 pounds skinless chicken thighs

1 tablespoon finely chopped fresh thyme

⅓ cup low-sodium chicken broth

Zest of 1 lime

2 garlic cloves, minced

2 teaspoons extra-virgin olive oil

1 teaspoon freshly ground black pepper

½ teaspoon salt

1 lemon, sliced

3 to 4 thyme sprigs

1. Spread the onion in the bottom of the slow cooker, and place the chicken thighs on top.

2. In a medium bowl, mix the chopped fresh thyme, broth, lime zest, garlic, olive oil, pepper, and salt. Pour the sauce over the chicken, and top with a layer of lemon slices.

3. Cook on low for 5 to 7 hours.

4. Garnish with springs of fresh thyme and serve.

COOKING TIP: Double the sauce and you can make this dish using a whole chicken. Check that the chicken will fit, though; you may need a larger slow cooker.

PER SERVING Calories: 294; Total Fat: 11g; Saturated Fat: 2g; Cholesterol: 190mg; Sodium: 398mg; Potassium: 44mg; Carbs: 3g; Fiber: 1g; Protein: 45g

Chicken Fajitas

LOWER SODIUM

ALLERGY-FRIENDLY • GLUTEN-FREE • LOW-CARB

Store-bought seasonings contain high levels of sodium. Making your own homemade seasoning blend eliminates that problem. Ditch the packet and use my Homemade Fajita Blend. The same goes for salsa, which can be loaded with salt, sugar, and thickeners. Make it yourself with just a few simple ingredients.

2½ cups Salsa (page 29)

2 pounds boneless, skinless chicken breasts, sliced

1 onion, sliced

2 bell peppers, seeded and sliced

2 tablespoons Homemade Fajita Blend (page 8)

1. Spread the salsa over the bottom of the slow cooker. Add the chicken, onion, bell peppers, and fajita blend, and stir to mix well.
2. Cook on low for 4 to 6 hours and serve.

VARIATION: You can substitute sliced flank steak, pork shoulder, or another meat for the chicken.

PER SERVING Calories: 201; Total Fat: 2g; Saturated Fat: 1g; Cholesterol: 88mg; Sodium: 167mg; Potassium: 543mg; Carbs: 8g; Fiber: 2g; Protein: 36g

Chicken Enchiladas

SERVES 6 • **PREP TIME:** 15 MINUTES • **COOK TIME:** 3 TO 4 HOURS ON LOW

LOW SODIUM

LOW-CARB

If you're looking to use up some leftover chicken thigh or breast meat, this recipe is for you. Corn tortillas keep this dish gluten-free, but use flour ones if you prefer. The green chiles in this recipe come from either a can or a jar. You should be able to find them easily in your local grocery. Look for products with no added ingredients.

Nonstick cooking spray

2½ pounds boneless, skinless chicken, cooked and shredded

½ cup Salsa (page 29)

3 cups Enchilada Sauce (page 28), divided

½ cup diced green chiles

12 (6-inch) corn tortillas

2 cups shredded low-fat Cheddar cheese

Handful chopped fresh cilantro

1. Spray the slow cooker generously with nonstick cooking spray.
2. In a large bowl, mix together the chicken, salsa, and ½ cup of enchilada sauce.
3. In a medium bowl, mix together the remaining 2½ cups of enchilada sauce and the green chiles.
4. Put ¼ cup of the chicken mixture on a tortilla. Roll the tortilla and place it seam-side down in the bottom of the slow cooker. You will need to lay the enchiladas down in layers in the slow cooker. Top each layer with a spoonful of enchilada sauce and some cheese. Repeat until all the tortillas are used.
5. Cook on low for 3 to 4 hours.
6. Garnish with cilantro before serving.

COOING TIP: Top your finished enchiladas with low-fat sour cream, avocados, more salsa, more cheese, shredded lettuce, and whatever else you like.

PER SERVING Calories: 546; Total Fat: 29g; Saturated Fat: 12g; Cholesterol: 176mg; Sodium: 463mg; Potassium: 941mg; Carbs: 20g; Fiber: 4g; Protein: 52g

Chicken and Corn Chowder Casserole

SERVES 6 • **PREP TIME:** 10 MINUTES • **COOK TIME:** 4 TO 6 HOURS ON LOW

LOW SODIUM

LOW-CARB

This is another recipe that conveniently uses leftover chicken. Most chicken and corn casseroles contain some sort of canned cream of something soup. Cream soups, like cream of mushroom, are usually high-sodium, so I've replaced it here with a combination of cheeses, butter, and milk.

1 pound skinless, boneless chicken, cooked and diced

2 (15-ounce) cans corn, drained and rinsed

1 bell pepper, seeded and diced

6 ounces low-fat cream cheese, cut into pieces

¼ cup unsalted butter, cut into pieces

¾ cup low-fat milk or almond milk

¾ cup shredded low-fat Cheddar cheese

1 tablespoon honey

¼ teaspoon salt

¼ teaspoon freshly ground black pepper

1. In the slow cooker, combine the chicken, corn, bell pepper, cream cheese, butter, milk, Cheddar, honey, salt, and pepper. Stir to mix well.
2. Cook on low for 4 to 6 hours and serve.

VARIATION: Depending on how hearty you want to go, you can stir up to 8 ounces of cooked pasta into the finished dish.

PER SERVING Calories: 391; Total Fat: 21g; Saturated Fat: 10g; Cholesterol: 95mg; Sodium: 491mg; Potassium: 254mg; Carbs: 25g; Fiber: 3g; Protein: 27g

Cajun Chicken and Potatoes

SERVES 6 • **PREP TIME:** 10 MINUTES • **COOK TIME:** 5 TO 7 HOURS ON LOW

LOW SODIUM

LOW-CARB

Cajun spices in a homemade sauce cook with chicken and potatoes in this super easy, healthy, and flavorful slow cooker dish. This is great served with a simple salad or a side of green vegetables, such as green beans, broccoli, or Brussels sprouts.

2 pounds skinless chicken

1 pound red potatoes or sweet potatoes, quartered

1 onion, sliced

3 celery stalks, chopped

1 bell pepper, seeded and chopped

⅓ cup water

2 tablespoons low-sodium soy sauce (or tamari if gluten-free)

2 tablespoons apple cider vinegar

2 tablespoons Homemade Cajun Blend (page 8)

2 teaspoons honey

2 garlic cloves, minced

1 teaspoon extra-virgin olive oil

¼ teaspoon salt

¼ teaspoon freshly ground black pepper

1. In the slow cooker, combine the chicken, potatoes, onion, celery, and bell pepper. Stir to mix well.
2. In a medium bowl, whisk together the water, soy sauce, vinegar, Cajun blend, honey, garlic, olive oil, salt, and pepper. Pour the sauce over the ingredients in the slow cooker.
3. Cook on low for 5 to 7 hours and serve.

VARIATION: Turn this into a hearty stew with gravy by adding 2 cups of chicken broth.

PER SERVING Calories: 271; Total Fat: 6g; Saturated Fat: 2g; Cholesterol: 87mg; Sodium: 490mg; Potassium: 440mg; Carbs: 18g; Fiber: 2g; Protein: 36g

Chicken with Apples and Potatoes

SERVES 4 • **PREP TIME:** 10 MINUTES • **COOK TIME:** 5 TO 7 HOURS ON LOW

LOW SODIUM

Chicken, apples, and potatoes may seem like an unlikely trio, but trust me, they go well together! This one-pot meal is satisfying without being too heavy. Since apples are a firm fruit, they hold up well during the low and slow cooking process. They also provide a touch of sweetness to the dish.

1 pound potatoes, quartered

1 small onion, sliced

1 pound apples, sliced, divided

1½ pounds skinless chicken legs or thighs

⅓ cup honey

¼ cup apple cider vinegar

2 tablespoons low-sodium soy sauce (or tamari if gluten-free)

½ teaspoon ground cinnamon

¼ teaspoon ground cumin

1. Put the potatoes, onion, and about half of the sliced apples in the bottom of the slow cooker. Stir to mix well, and scatter the chicken on top.

2. In a small bowl, mix together the honey, vinegar, soy sauce, cinnamon, and cumin. Pour the sauce into the slow cooker, coating all the ingredients.

3. Top with the remaining apples.

4. Cook on low for 5 to 7 hours and serve.

INGREDIENT TIP: Sweet apple or tart? That's up to you. You can even do a mix of both. Gala and Red Delicious are my favorite sweet apples, while my go-to tart apple is Granny Smith.

PER SERVING Calories: 434; Total Fat: 2g; Saturated Fat: 1g; Cholesterol: 99mg; Sodium: 386mg; Potassium: 1,088mg; Carbs: 61g; Fiber: 4g; Protein: 43g

Coconut-Curry Chicken

SERVES 4 • **PREP TIME:** 5 MINUTES • **COOK TIME:** 4 TO 6 HOURS ON LOW

LOW SODIUM

ALLERGY-FRIENDLY • GLUTEN-FREE • LOW-CARB

Curry is another dish that's perfect for the slow cooker because the longer the ingredients cook in the broth of coconut milk, the more powerful the flavors. Asian ingredients slowly cook with chicken in this heavily aromatic yet simple slow cooker curry. Use full-fat coconut milk for a creamier curry, or light coconut milk if you're watching your calories. Chicken thighs work better in curries, in my opinion, but you can absolutely substitute breasts if you prefer.

1½ pounds boneless, skinless chicken thighs

1 (15-ounce) can full-fat or light coconut milk

3 large carrots, chopped

1 onion, chopped

4 garlic cloves, minced

1 tablespoon curry powder

1 teaspoon red pepper flakes

1 teaspoon ground ginger

½ teaspoon salt

½ teaspoon ground coriander

¼ teaspoon freshly ground black pepper

¼ cup chopped fresh cilantro

1. In the slow cooker, combine the chicken, coconut milk, carrots, onion, garlic, curry powder, red pepper flakes, ginger, salt, coriander, and pepper. Stir to mix well.

2. Cook on low for 4 to 6 hours.

3. Garnish with fresh cilantro and serve.

INGREDIENT TIP: Coconut fat is a saturated fat, but a special kind called medium-chain saturated fatty acids (MCFAs). Unlike other kinds of saturated fats, MCFAs are metabolized more quickly by the body and are less likely to be stored as fat.

PER SERVING Calories: 486; Total Fat: 33g; Saturated Fat: 24g; Cholesterol: 143mg; Sodium: 496mg; Potassium: 546mg; Carbs: 16g; Fiber: 5g; Protein: 37g

Chili-Lime Chicken

SERVES 4 • **PREP TIME:** 5 MINUTES • **COOK TIME:** 4 TO 6 HOURS ON LOW

LOW SODIUM

ALLERGY-FRIENDLY • LOW-CARB

Succulent, shredded chili-lime chicken can be served as a taco or enchilada filling, in a tortilla, over rice, in a salad, as a stuffing for stuffed peppers—the possibilities are endless. You don't even have to shred the chicken. Leave the breasts whole and serve them over rice or mashed potatoes. Please note, this dish uses just one chipotle chile in adobo, not the entire can.

1 pound boneless, skinless chicken breasts

1 small onion, diced

2 garlic cloves, minced

1 tablespoon honey

1 chipotle chile in adobo, chopped

1 teaspoon ground cumin

1 teaspoon dried oregano

1 teaspoon paprika

¼ teaspoon salt

¼ teaspoon ground cinnamon

⅓ cup Enchilada Sauce (page 28)

Juice of 2 limes

¼ cup water, if needed

⅓ cup chopped fresh cilantro

1. In the slow cooker, combine the chicken, onion, garlic, honey, chile, cumin, oregano, paprika, salt, cinnamon, enchilada sauce, and lime juice. Stir to mix well.
2. Cook on low for 4 to 6 hours.
3. When the chicken is done, transfer to a plate and shred with two forks. Return it to the slow cooker and heat through.
4. If the sauce is too thick, stir in the water.
5. Garnish with fresh cilantro and serve.

INGREDIENT TIP: Chipotle chiles in adobo are spicy chipotle peppers marinated in a red sauce, which brings out more of their wonderful smoky and spicy flavor. A little bit really does go a long way with these chiles, so you won't need much. And be careful with the red sauce; it packs a punch, too.

PER SERVING Calories: 169; Total Fat: 2g; Saturated Fat: 0g; Cholesterol: 65mg; Sodium: 343mg; Potassium: 97mg; Carbs: 11g; Fiber: 2g; Protein: 27g

Cashew Chicken

SERVES 4 • **PREP TIME:** 10 MINUTES • **COOK TIME:** 4 HOURS 15 MINUTES
TO 6 HOURS 20 MINUTES ON LOW

LOW SODIUM

Never eat takeout cashew chicken again! Cashew chicken is a traditional American-Chinese dish that's not known for being especially healthy. But the basic ingredients—cashews, chicken, and veggies—all are. It's the added salt, MSG, and oil that give this dish a bad reputation. Making it at home eliminates all the bad and keeps all the good.

1 pound boneless, skinless chicken breasts, cut into 1-inch pieces

1 cup chopped unsalted cashews

2 cups carrots, peeled and finely chopped

2 cups chopped broccoli

¼ cup low-sodium soy sauce (or tamari if gluten-free)

¾ cup no-salt-added chicken broth

⅓ cup rice wine vinegar

⅓ cup Ketchup (page 25)

2 tablespoons honey

2 garlic cloves, minced

2 teaspoons ground ginger

¼ teaspoon red pepper flakes

Freshly ground black pepper

¼ cup water

2 tablespoons cornstarch

1. In the slow cooker, combine the chicken, cashews, carrots, broccoli, soy sauce, chicken broth, vinegar, ketchup, honey, garlic, ginger, and red pepper flakes, and season lightly with pepper. Stir to mix well.

2. Cook on low for 4 to 6 hours.

3. In a small bowl, mix together the water with the cornstarch. Pour the slurry into the slow cooker and stir.

4. Cook for an additional 15 to 20 minutes, or until the sauce has thickened, and serve.

COOKING TIP: Serve this chicken over brown rice, or better yet, stir a couple cups of cooked brown rice directly into the slow cooker after the cooking is done.

PER SERVING Calories: 441; Total Fat: 18g; Saturated Fat: 3g; Cholesterol: 65mg; Sodium: 531mg; Potassium: 539mg; Carbs: 37g; Fiber: 3g; Protein: 37g

Spicy Piri-Piri Chicken

SERVES 6 • **PREP TIME:** 10 MINUTES • **COOK TIME:** 4 TO 6 HOURS ON LOW

LOW SODIUM

ALLERGY-FRIENDLY • GLUTEN-FREE • LOW-CARB

Piri-piri chicken is a spicy chicken recipe created in North Africa when Portuguese settlers arrived with chile peppers (piri-piri in Swahili). It's spicy but not too overwhelming, so don't worry. To make this more of a complete meal, add 1 pound of chopped potatoes and a pound of vegetables, such as green beans, with the chicken at the start of cooking.

1 small onion, sliced

2 pounds skinless chicken parts

¼ cup freshly squeezed
  lemon juice

2 garlic cloves, minced

2 tablespoons white vinegar

1 tablespoon extra-virgin olive oil

2 teaspoons chili powder

2 teaspoons paprika

1 teaspoon ground
  cayenne pepper

1 teaspoon dried oregano

1 teaspoon ground ginger

½ teaspoon salt

½ teaspoon freshly ground
  black pepper

1 lemon, sliced

1. Place the sliced onion in the bottom of the slow cooker, and place the chicken on top.
2. In a medium bowl, mix together the lemon juice, garlic, vinegar, olive oil, chili powder, paprika, cayenne, oregano, ginger, salt, and pepper. Pour the sauce over chicken, and top with the lemon slices.
3. Cook on low for 4 to 6 hours and serve.

VARIATION: Rather than use a cut-up chicken, substitute a small, 2- to 3-pound whole chicken or even two Cornish hens.

PER SERVING Calories: 171; Total Fat: 6g; Saturated Fat: 2g; Cholesterol: 53mg; Sodium: 292mg; Potassium: 87mg; Carbs: 6g; Fiber: 1g; Protein: 25g

Chicken with Orzo and Lemon

SERVES 4 • **PREP TIME:** 10 MINUTES • **COOK TIME:** 5 TO 7 HOURS ON LOW

LOW SODIUM

When combined with more broth, chicken with orzo and lemon is actually a traditional Greek soup. This recipe has pretty much the same components, but in a casserole form. With a protein, grain, and vegetables, this is a true one-pot meal.

3 cups low-sodium chicken broth

1 cup uncooked orzo pasta

1 pound boneless, skinless chicken breasts

1 pound carrots, peeled and diced

1 small onion, diced

3 celery stalks diced

2 garlic cloves, minced

1 teaspoon dried thyme

1 teaspoon ground turmeric

½ teaspoon salt

½ teaspoon freshly ground black pepper

Juice of 1 lemon

2 dried bay leaves

2 tablespoons crumbled low-fat feta cheese (optional)

1. In the slow cooker, combine the broth, pasta, chicken, carrots, onion, celery, garlic, thyme, turmeric, salt, pepper, lemon juice, and bay leaves. Stir to mix well.
2. Cook on low for 5 to 7 hours.
3. Remove the bay leaves and top with the crumbled feta (if using) before serving.

VARIATION: Don't have thyme? Use rosemary or tarragon. Get creative with your herbs.

PER SERVING Calories: 288; Total Fat: 13g; Saturated Fat: 1g; Cholesterol: 84mg; Sodium: 467mg; Potassium: 541mg; Carbs: 30g; Fiber: 5g; Protein: 34g

Alfredo Pasta with Chicken

SERVES 6 • **PREP TIME:** 5 MINUTES • **COOK TIME:** 4 TO 6 HOURS ON LOW AND
20 TO 30 MINUTES ON HIGH

LOW SODIUM

Store-bought Alfredo sauces can be high in calories, fat, and sodium. Using the homemade Alfredo sauce in chapter 2 gives you more control over the nutritional value of the dish. In this creamy pasta recipe you can use your favorite type of pasta, whether it's penne, fettuccine, or linguine, whole-wheat or gluten-free.

2 pounds boneless, skinless chicken breasts

2 cups Alfredo Sauce (page 31)

1 small red onion, diced

2 garlic cloves, minced

1 teaspoon dried basil

1 teaspoon dried oregano

¼ teaspoon salt

¼ teaspoon freshly ground black pepper

8 ounces uncooked pasta

1. In the slow cooker, combine the chicken, Alfredo sauce, onion, garlic, basil, oregano, salt, and pepper. Stir to mix well.

2. Cook on low for 4 to 6 hours.

3. Add the pasta and stir until the noodles are completely coated and submerged in the sauce, with no pieces sticking out.

4. Cook for an additional 20 to 30 minutes on high, or until the pasta is tender, and serve immediately.

COOKING TIP: One of the keys to cooking pasta in the slow cooker is making sure there is enough liquid to cover it. Even with that in mind, you might want to keep an eye on the pasta and stir it very occasionally.

PER SERVING Calories: 448; Total Fat: 12g; Saturated Fat: 4g; Cholesterol: 101mg; Sodium: 398mg; Potassium: 442mg; Carbs: 35g; Fiber: 2g; Protein: 46g

Chicken and Dumplings

SERVES 6 • **PREP TIME:** 15 MINUTES • **COOK TIME:** 8 HOURS ON LOW

LOWER SODIUM

LOW-CARB

This is pretty much chicken soup with dumplings cooked on top. Store-bought dumpling/biscuit/pancake mixes are loaded with salt and chemicals. It's actually really easy to just make your own dumplings, and then you know exactly what's in them. In this recipe for homemade dumplings, I purposely didn't specify what type of flour to use, so you can decide whether you want to use whole-wheat, all-purpose, or gluten-free.

For the soup

1 pound cooked chicken, shredded

4 cups low-sodium chicken broth

½ cup frozen peas

1 onion, chopped

2 large carrots, peeled and chopped

2 celery stalks, chopped

1 teaspoon dried thyme

1 teaspoon garlic powder

Freshly ground black pepper

For the dumplings

1 cup flour

1 large egg, beaten

2 teaspoons baking powder

½ cup buttermilk

To make the soup

1. In the slow cooker, combine the chicken, broth, peas, onion, carrots, celery, thyme, and garlic powder, and season lightly with pepper. Stir to mix well.

2. Cook on low for 6 hours.

To make the dumplings

1. Just before 6 hours are done, in a medium bowl, mix together the flour, egg, baking powder, and buttermilk.

2. Scoop up ⅓ cup of the dumpling batter and place it in a ball on top of the soup. Repeat until you've added all the batter.

3. Cook on low for an additional 2 hours and serve.

VARIATION: Get creative and add your favorite diced vegetables to the soup before cooking.

PER SERVING Calories: 251; Total Fat: 4g; Saturated Fat: 1g; Cholesterol: 86mg; Sodium: 159mg; Potassium: 512mg; Carbs: 25g; Fiber: 3g; Protein: 28g

Turkey Breast with Apple Cider Gravy

SERVES 4 TO 6 • **PREP TIME:** 5 MINUTES • **COOK TIME:** 5 TO 7 HOURS ON LOW

LOW SODIUM

ALLERGY-FRIENDLY • LOW-CARB

The touch of apples and cider provides a unique sweet and tangy spin to this turkey breast recipe. Using a simple homemade gravy that can also be made in the slow cooker makes this dish not only healthier but a lot more flavorful, too.

2 cups Gravy (page 26)

¼ cup apple cider vinegar

1 teaspoon ground cinnamon

¼ teaspoon salt

½ teaspoon ground cumin

¼ teaspoon freshly ground black pepper

2 to 3 pounds whole boneless turkey breast

½ cup low-sodium chicken broth

1. In the bottom of the slow cooker, mix to combine the gravy, vinegar, cinnamon, salt, cumin, and pepper.

2. Add the turkey breast, then pour the broth on top.

3. Cook on low for 5 to 7 hours and serve.

VARIATION: You can make this recipe with chicken. Substitute 2 to 3 pounds of boneless, skinless breasts for the turkey.

PER SERVING Calories: 438; Total Fat: 4g; Saturated Fat: 0g; Cholesterol: 210mg; Sodium: 363mg; Potassium: 1,028mg; Carbs: 5g; Fiber: 0g; Protein: 84g

Broccoli Slaw-ghetti with Ground Turkey

SERVES 4 • **PREP TIME:** 5 MINUTES • **COOK TIME:** 5 TO 6 HOURS ON LOW

LOWER SODIUM

ALLERGY-FRIENDLY • GLUTEN-FREE • LOW-CARB

Slaw-ghetti is broccoli slaw cooked in the slow cooker to a soft, spaghetti-like consistency. This is a great low-carb alternative to spaghetti that's not spaghetti squash. You should be able to find pre-made broccoli slaw in the produce section of your local supermarket. If not, you can make your own by peeling and thinly slicing or shredding 5 or 6 large broccoli stems and 1 or 2 medium carrots.

12 ounces broccoli slaw

1 pound ground turkey, browned

1 (24-ounce) can no-salt-added
  diced tomatoes

1 bell pepper, seeded and sliced

2 garlic cloves, minced

¼ cup chopped spinach

2 teaspoons Homemade Italian
  Blend (page 9)

Chopped fresh parsley,
  for garnish

1. In the slow cooker, combine the broccoli slaw, turkey, tomatoes and their juices, bell pepper, garlic, spinach, and Italian blend. Stir to mix well.
2. Cook on low for 5 to 6 hours, or until the broccoli slaw is soft.
3. Top with chopped fresh parsley and serve.

VARIATION: Add your favorite vegetables, such as diced onion and mushrooms. I like spinach here, but kale, collard greens, and Swiss chard are possibilities. Also consider adding your favorite fresh herbs.

PER SERVING Calories: 241; Total Fat: 10g; Saturated Fat: 3g; Cholesterol: 90mg; Sodium: 145mg; Potassium: 1,009mg; Carbs: 15g; Fiber: 5g; Protein: 24g

Turkey Burger Casserole

SERVES 4 TO 6 • **PREP TIME:** 10 MINUTES • **COOK TIME:** 3 TO 5 HOURS ON LOW,
PLUS 10 MINUTES ON THE STOVE TOP

LOW SODIUM

ALLERGY-FRIENDLY • GLUTEN-FREE

This kid-friendly casserole has the essence of a turkey burger and fries, but in a casserole form. This can also be a freezer meal—after all, it starts with frozen sweet potatoes. Make your own fries if you don't want to use frozen. Just cut some fresh potatoes or sweet potatoes into thick wedges.

1½ pounds ground turkey

1 (28-ounce) can no-salt-added diced tomatoes

1 medium onion, chopped

2 bell peppers, seeded and chopped

2 garlic cloves, minced

2 tablespoons mustard

½ teaspoon salt

½ teaspoon freshly ground black pepper

1 tablespoon relish (optional)

10 to 12 ounces frozen sweet potato fries

1. In a large skillet over medium heat, cook the ground turkey until browned, about 10 minutes. Drain off any excess fat. Add the tomatoes and their juices, onion, bell pepper, garlic, mustard, salt, pepper, and relish (if using) to the skillet. Stir to mix well.

2. Add the mixture to the slow cooker, and top with a layer of frozen fries.

3. Cook on low for 3 to 5 hours and serve.

INGREDIENT TIP: Sweet potatoes not only have more fiber and more complex carbohydrates than white potatoes, they're one of the best sources of vitamin A, which is good for your immune system.

PER SERVING Calories: 402; Total Fat: 11g; Saturated Fat: 1g; Cholesterol: 93mg; Sodium: 472mg; Potassium: 1,152mg; Carbs: 35g; Fiber: 7g; Protein: 45g

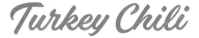

Turkey Chili

SERVES 4 TO 6 • **PREP TIME:** 10 MINUTES • **COOK TIME:** 4 TO 6 HOURS ON LOW, PLUS 10 MINUTES ON THE STOVE TOP

LOW SODIUM

ALLERGY-FRIENDLY • GLUTEN-FREE

Chili is made to be cooked in the slow cooker. This is a simple dish of ground turkey, kidney beans, tomatoes, and seasonings. Of course, you can use ground beef, chicken, or even pork in place of the ground turkey. And like most chilis, it's better the next day!

2 pounds ground turkey or turkey sausage

1 (28-ounce) can no-salt-added crushed tomatoes

1 (10-ounce) can no-salt-added diced tomatoes with green chiles

1 cup Marinara Sauce (page 30)

1 (15-ounce) can red kidney beans, drained and rinsed

1 onion, chopped

3 garlic cloves, minced

2 tablespoons chili powder

2 teaspoons ground cumin

1½ teaspoons paprika

¼ teaspoon salt

1 teaspoon dried oregano

1. In a large skillet over medium heat, cook the ground meat or sausage until browned, about 12 minutes. Drain the fat, and transfer the meat to the slow cooker.

2. Add the crushed tomatoes and diced tomatoes with chiles and their juices, marinara sauce, beans, onion, garlic, chili powder, cumin, paprika, salt, and oregano to the slow cooker. Stir to mix well.

3. Cook on low for 4 to 6 hours and serve.

INGREDIENT TIP: Some store-bought turkey sausages can have just as much sodium as regular sausages. Look for an uncured, reduced-sodium brand that's nitrate-free.

PER SERVING Calories: 456; Total Fat: 9g; Saturated Fat: 1g; Cholesterol: 87mg; Sodium: 487mg; Potassium: 427mg; Carbs: 45g; Fiber: 15g; Protein: 49g

Turkey Tetrazzini

SERVES 4 • **PREP TIME:** 15 MINUTES • **COOK TIME:** 4 HOURS 15 MINUTES TO 6 HOURS 15 MINUTES ON LOW, PLUS 45 MINUTES TO ROAST AND 5 MINUTES ON THE STOVE TOP

LOW SODIUM

GLUTEN-FREE • LOW-CARB

I don't know about you but whenever I cook a whole turkey, I have tons left over and I don't know what to do with them. Here's a recipe that uses some of that leftover turkey. This is a low-carb version of turkey tetrazzini that uses spaghetti squash in place of pasta and a light, cheesy yet healthy homemade sauce.

2 pounds spaghetti squash, cooked

1 pound cooked turkey, diced

1 small onion, diced

½ cup sliced mushrooms

3 garlic cloves, minced

1 teaspoon garlic powder

¼ teaspoon salt

½ teaspoon ground cumin

¾ teaspoon freshly ground black pepper, divided

½ teaspoon dried sage

½ teaspoon dried parsley

¼ teaspoon celery salt

1 tablespoon unsalted butter

1 tablespoon almond flour

¾ cup low-fat milk

1 cup low-fat mozzarella cheese, divided

2 tablespoons grated Parmesan cheese

1. Preheat the oven to 400°F.

2. Halve the squash, and scrape out the seeds. Lay the squash halves cut-side down on a roasting pan and cook for 30 to 45 minutes, until tender when pierced with a fork. Cool slightly.

3. Shred the spaghetti squash with a fork. Add the squash strands, turkey, onion, mushrooms, garlic, garlic powder, salt, cumin, ½ teaspoon of pepper, sage, parsley, and celery salt to the slow cooker. Stir to mix well.

4. In a medium saucepan over medium heat, melt the butter. Whisk in the almond flour, and heat until bubbling. Slowly pour in the milk, whisking the entire time, until blended. Add the remaining ¼ teaspoon of pepper. Slowly add in ½ cup of mozzarella cheese, stirring the entire time. Whisk until the cheese is melted, a few minutes.

5. Pour the sauce mixture into the slow cooker, and stir again to mix well. Top with the Parmesan cheese.

6. Cook on low for 4 to 6 hours.

7. Sprinkle the remaining ½ cup of mozzarella cheese over the top, and cook for an additional 15 minutes on low, until the cheese melts, and serve.

VARIATION: If you're not following a low-carb lifestyle, you can substitute 8 ounces of cooked pasta for the spaghetti squash.

PER SERVING Calories: 384; Total Fat: 14g; Saturated Fat: 7g; Cholesterol: 107mg; Sodium: 443mg; Potassium: 734mg; Carbs: 22g; Fiber: 1g; Protein: 42g

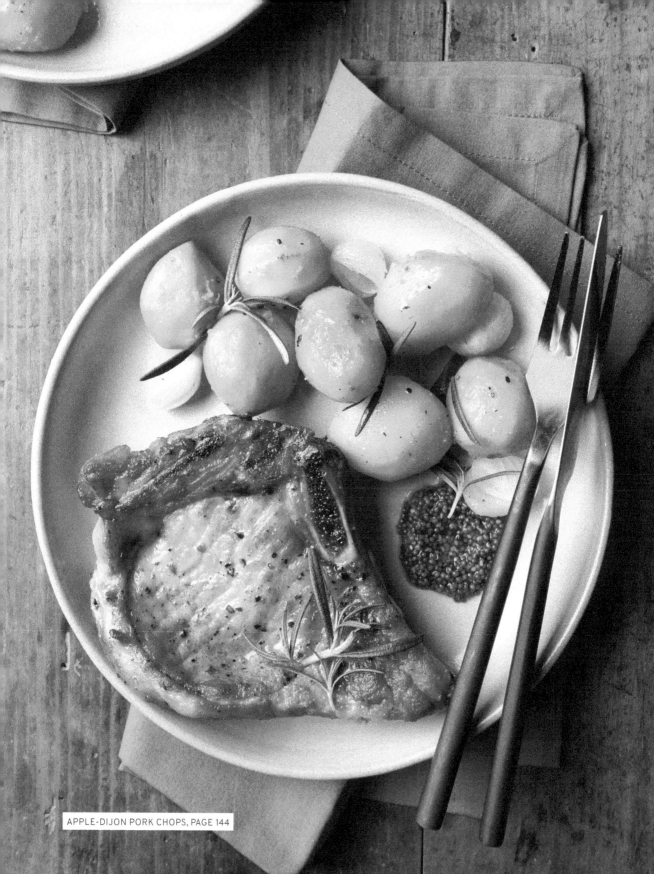

APPLE-DIJON PORK CHOPS, PAGE 144

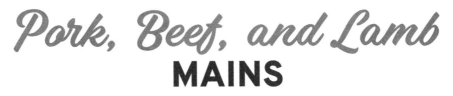

Pork, Beef, and Lamb
MAINS

Herbed Pork Loin

SERVES 4 • **PREP TIME:** 5 MINUTES • **COOK TIME:** 6 TO 8 HOURS ON LOW

LOW SODIUM

ALLERGY-FRIENDLY • LOW-CARB

Fresh herbs and a light, homemade, creamy sauce cook together in this recipe, which might look fancy but is really simple. The pork loin cooks whole, so you can slice or even shred the meat when it's done cooking.

2 to 3 pounds whole pork loin

1 cup low-sodium chicken broth

1 tablespoon melted unsalted butter or extra-virgin olive oil

2 garlic cloves, minced

1 teaspoon dried parsley

1 teaspoon dried oregano

1 teaspoon dried basil

1 teaspoon dried thyme

¼ teaspoon garlic powder

¼ teaspoon salt

¼ teaspoon freshly ground black pepper

1. Place the pork in the bottom of the slow cooker.
2. In a medium bowl, mix together the broth, butter, garlic, parsley, oregano, basil, thyme, garlic powder, salt, and pepper. Pour the sauce on top of the pork.
3. Cook on low for 6 to 8 hours and serve.

INGREDIENT TIP: Fresh herbs have more flavor than dried, so use them if you have them! Be sure to use the proper conversion, which is three times more fresh herbs than dry.

PER SERVING Calories: 799; Total Fat: 58g; Saturated Fat: 22g; Cholesterol: 280mg; Sodium: 421mg; Potassium: 1,460mg; Carbs: 1g; Fiber: 0g; Protein: 68g

Filipino Pork Adobo

SERVES 6 • **PREP TIME:** 5 MINUTES • **COOK TIME:** 6 TO 8 HOURS ON LOW

LOW SODIUM

LOW-CARB

Pork adobo is a traditional Filipino recipe. And like most traditional recipes, there are tons of variations out there. This is a cleaned-up version that eliminates sugar and uses reduced-sodium soy sauce (or tamari, if gluten is a concern for you). The pork cooks until it's falling-apart tender. Serve this over cauliflower rice or brown rice or with potatoes.

3 pounds pork shoulder, cut into chunks

2 tablespoons low-sodium soy sauce (or tamari if gluten-free)

4 garlic cloves, minced

1½ cups low-sodium beef broth

4 dried bay leaves

1 teaspoon oyster sauce

2 teaspoons whole peppercorns

¼ cup apple cider vinegar

1½ teaspoons honey

Freshly ground black pepper

1. In the slow cooker, combine the pork, soy sauce, garlic, broth, bay leaves, oyster sauce, peppercorns, vinegar, and honey, and season with pepper. Stir to mix well.

2. Cook on low for 6 to 8 hours, or until the pork is tender.

3. Remove the bay leaves before serving.

INGREDIENT TIP: Oyster sauce is made with salt, sugar, cornstarch, and yes, oyster essence. You'll find it with the Asian foods in your supermarket. The wrong oyster sauce can also be loaded with sodium and MSG. Make sure to read the nutritional values on the back of the bottle before purchasing.

PER SERVING Calories: 368; Total Fat: 12g; Saturated Fat: 4g; Cholesterol: 173mg; Sodium: 496mg; Potassium: 17mg; Carbs: 3g; Fiber: 0g; Protein: 58g

Apple-Dijon Pork Chops

SERVES 4 • **PREP TIME:** 10 MINUTES • **COOK TIME:** 6 TO 8 HOURS ON LOW

LOWER SODIUM

ALLERGY-FRIENDLY • LOW-CARB

Homemade applesauce adds a unique spin to this pork chop recipe, and its sweetness balances the mustard and vinegar. This recipe can serve as a kind of template for other dishes. Try it with thick slices of turkey breast or skinless chicken thighs.

1 pound potatoes, whole

1 small onion, sliced

1 cup Applesauce (page 34)

Salt

Freshly ground black pepper

1½ pounds boneless pork chops

2 tablespoons fresh or
  1 tablespoon dried rosemary

3 garlic cloves, minced

2 tablespoons Dijon mustard

2 tablespoons apple cider vinegar

¾ cup low-sodium chicken broth

Chopped fresh rosemary, for
  garnish (optional)

Red peppercorns, for garnish
  (optional)

Fresh sage, for garnish (optional)

1. Put the potatoes, onion, and applesauce in the bottom of the slow cooker, and season lightly with salt and pepper. Stir to mix well. Arrange the pork chops on top.

2. In a medium bowl, whisk together the rosemary, garlic, mustard, vinegar, and broth. Pour the sauce on top of the other ingredients in the slow cooker.

3. Cook on low for 6 to 8 hours.

4. Top with fresh rosemary, peppercorns, and sage (if using) before serving.

COOKING TIP: You can substitute one large apple that's been diced finely for the applesauce.

PER SERVING Calories: 334; Total Fat: 7g; Saturated Fat: 2g; Cholesterol: 113mg; Sodium: 233mg; Potassium: 558mg; Carbs: 28g; Fiber: 4g; Protein: 41g

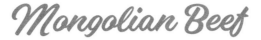

Mongolian Beef

SERVES 4 • **PREP TIME:** 5 MINUTES • **COOK TIME:** 4 TO 6 HOURS ON LOW

LOW SODIUM

LOW-CARB

Homemade Mongolian beef is obviously way healthier than takeout, because you use fresh ingredients and a homemade sauce. This version is simple to make, and it will also work well with skinless chicken thighs. Serve the finished meal over rice or cauliflower rice.

1½ pounds skirt or flank steak, sliced

1 cup water

¼ cup low-sodium soy sauce (or tamari if gluten-free)

⅓ cup honey

2 garlic cloves, minced

3 green onions, finely chopped

1. In the slow cooker, combine the steak, water, soy sauce, honey, and garlic. Stir to mix well.

2. Cook on low for 4 to 6 hours.

3. Garnish with the green onions just before serving.

COOKING TIP: To thicken up the sauce after the dish is cooked, mix together 2 tablespoons of water and ¼ cup of cornstarch and slowly stir it into the slow cooker. Heat until the sauce is thickened to your liking.

PER SERVING Calories: 357; Total Fat: 14g; Saturated Fat: 5g; Cholesterol: 68mg; Sodium: 350mg; Potassium: 436mg; Carbs: 27g; Fiber: 1g; Protein: 32g

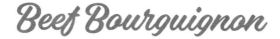

Beef Bourguignon

SERVES 4 • **PREP TIME:** 10 MINUTES • **COOK TIME:** 6 TO 8 HOURS ON LOW

LOW SODIUM

ALLERGY-FRIENDLY • GLUTEN-FREE

Anyone else think of Julia Child when cooking bourguignon? This French classic comes from the Burgundy region and is traditionally made by braising beef in red wine and broth with garlic, onions, and mushrooms. Lardons (strips of pork fat) made the meat tender. It's a dish that's perfect for the slow cooker, which produces extremely tender beef—without the lardons or the wine. You would never guess this meal is healthy because the flavor is so rich, but at the end of the day, basically it's just meat and vegetables.

3 pounds beef stew meat

4 cups Beef Bone Broth (page 24)

⅓ pound low-sodium bacon, cooked and crumbled

8 ounces sliced mushrooms

1½ pounds carrots, peeled and chopped

1 pound baby potatoes

1 large onion, chopped

4 garlic cloves, minced

2 dried bay leaves

Salt

Freshly ground black pepper

¼ cup chopped fresh parsley

1. In the slow cooker, combine the stew meat, broth, bacon, mushrooms, carrots, potatoes, onion, garlic, and bay leaves, and season lightly with salt and pepper. Stir to mix well.

2. Cook on low for 6 to 8 hours.

3. Remove the bay leaves and top with fresh parsley before serving.

VARIATION: For a more authentic French flavor, substitute one bottle of red wine for the broth.

PER SERVING Calories: 661; Total Fat: 26g; Saturated Fat: 5g; Cholesterol: 30mg; Sodium: 437mg; Potassium: 1,550mg; Carbs: 37g; Fiber: 9g; Protein: 87g

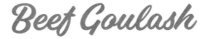

Beef Goulash

SERVES 6 • **PREP TIME:** 10 MINUTES • **COOK TIME:** 6 TO 8 HOURS ON LOW

LOWER SODIUM

ALLERGY-FRIENDLY • LOW-CARB • LOW-CHOLESTEROL

Goulash is a traditional Hungarian stew made from chunks of meat slow cooked in a mixture of paprika, tomatoes, and other vegetables. It's traditionally cooked with tough cuts of meat that become tender through long, low, moist cooking—perfect for the slow cooker. As with most traditional recipes, there are a lot of different versions out there. This low-sodium version one doesn't cut any corners on flavor.

2 pounds beef stew meat

1 large onion, diced

3 celery stalks, diced

1 bell pepper, seeded and diced

1 (28-ounce) can no-salt-added diced tomatoes

2½ cups low-sodium beef broth

2 garlic cloves, minced

2 tablespoons no-salt-added tomato purée

2 tablespoons paprika

1 teaspoon ground cumin

Salt

Freshly ground black pepper

1. In the slow cooker, combine the stew meat, onion, celery, bell pepper, tomatoes and their juices, broth, garlic, tomato purée, paprika, and cumin, and season lightly with salt and pepper. Stir to mix well.

2. Cook on low for 6 to 8 hours and serve.

VARIATION: Turn this into a hearty soup by adding an additional 4 cups of beef broth.

PER SERVING Calories: 277; Total Fat: 10g; Saturated Fat: 0g; Cholesterol: 50mg; Sodium: 102mg; Potassium: 502mg; Carbs: 12g; Fiber: 4g; Protein: 36g

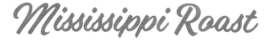

Mississippi Roast

SERVES 6 • **PREP TIME:** 5 MINUTES • **COOK TIME:** 8 TO 9 HOURS ON LOW

LOWER SODIUM

ALLERGY-FRIENDLY • GLUTEN-FREE • LOW-CARB

Mississippi Roast is a classic slow cooker recipe that typically includes a packet of ranch dressing mix, sometimes a packet of dry onion soup, and up to a stick of butter! But you can throw away the store-bought seasoning and cut way back on the butter. While this is a much healthier version of the Mississippi roast, it's not lacking the flavor that made this recipe famous in the first place.

1 (3-pound) chuck roast

2 tablespoons Homemade Dry Onion Soup Mix (page 9)

2 tablespoons Homemade Dry Ranch Dressing Mix (page 9)

8 pepperoncini peppers, fresh or jarred

2 to 4 tablespoons unsalted butter (or ghee, if allergy-friendly)

1. Place the whole roast in the bottom of the slow cooker, and sprinkle the homemade dry mixes on top. Add the pepperoncinis and butter on top of the dry spices.

2. Cook on low for 8 to 9 hours and serve.

COOKING TIP: You'll know it's done when the meat is so tender it shreds with a fork. In fact, it's best served shredded, rather than slicing the roast whole.

PER SERVING Calories: 398; Total Fat: 19g; Saturated Fat: 9g; Cholesterol: 143mg; Sodium: 171mg; Potassium: 860mg; Carbs: 3g; Fiber: 1g; Protein: 50g

Lamb Shanks and Cabbage

SERVES 4 • **PREP TIME:** 5 MINUTES • **COOK TIME:** 6 TO 8 HOURS ON LOW

LOW SODIUM

ALLERGY-FRIENDLY

Lamb shanks seems like one of those impossibly fancy dishes you can only get at a restaurant. The shank is the shin—the bone and meat below the knee. It's a tough cut, so it must cook long and low anyway. The bone is full of flavor, and also collagen, which will naturally thicken the gravy. Impress your friends with this very simple recipe; really, you're just throwing all the ingredients in the slow cooker and letting it do its magic. Serve this over egg noodles, rice, or mashed potatoes.

2 pounds lamb shanks

1 cup low-sodium beef broth

1 medium head cabbage, cored and chopped

1½ pounds potatoes, chopped

1 onion, chopped

2 garlic cloves, minced

1 teaspoon ground cumin

½ teaspoon salt

½ teaspoon freshly ground black pepper

1. In the slow cooker, combine the lamb, broth, cabbage, potatoes, onion, garlic, cumin, salt, and pepper. Stir to mix well.
2. Cook on low for 6 to 8 hours and serve.

INGREDIENT TIP: Lamb shanks can be expensive. A cheaper alternative is lamb neck bones.

PER SERVING Calories: 611; Total Fat: 27g; Saturated Fat: 12g; Cholesterol: 150mg; Sodium: 387mg; Potassium: 1,121mg; Carbs: 43g; Fiber: 10g; Protein: 51g

Lemon and Thyme Lamb Roast with Artichokes

SERVES 4 • **PREP TIME:** 10 MINUTES • **COOK TIME:** 6 TO 8 HOURS ON LOW

LOW SODIUM

ALLERGY-FRIENDLY • GLUTEN-FREE • LOW-CARB

Citrus and herbs combine for this colorful and healthy main dish. You can substitute a beef roast for the lamb without having to make any modifications to the recipe. As always, fresh herbs are better, so substitute 6 teaspoons of chopped fresh thyme if you can.

1 large onion, sliced

2-pound boneless lamb roast

2 lemons, sliced

1 (15-ounce) can water-packed artichokes, drained

4 garlic cloves, minced

¼ cup freshly squeezed lemon juice

1 tablespoon extra-virgin olive oil

2 teaspoons dried thyme

½ teaspoon salt

½ teaspoon freshly ground black pepper

1. Put the sliced onion in the slow cooker, and place the lamb, lemon slices, and artichokes on top.

2. In a small bowl, mix together the garlic, lemon juice, olive oil, thyme, salt, and pepper.

3. Pour the sauce into the slow cooker, making sure to coat all the ingredients.

4. Cook on low for 6 to 8 hours and serve.

INGREDIENT TIP: You don't need to fuss with fresh artichokes for this recipe; canned will work just fine. Be sure to drain them first, or go for frozen.

PER SERVING Calories: 705; Total Fat: 52g; Saturated Fat: 23g; Cholesterol: 160mg; Sodium: 467mg; Potassium: 487mg; Carbs: 17g; Fiber: 7g; Protein: 42g

North African Lamb

SERVES 4 • PREP TIME: 10 MINUTES • COOK TIME: 6 TO 8 HOURS ON LOW

LOWER SODIUM

ALLERGY-FRIENDLY • LOW-CARB

The aroma of North Africa will overtake your kitchen with this easy yet impressive recipe. You can use whatever cut of lamb you like—shoulder, leg, shanks, stew, or even rack of lamb. Lamb can be expensive, but this versatile dish means you can pick a cheaper cut. Personally, I prefer a boneless cut, but it's up to you. Make this a complete meal by adding 1 pound of chopped potatoes at the start of cooking, or serve over rice or couscous with vegetables on the side.

¼ cup low-sodium beef broth or water

2 pounds lamb shoulder

½ pound carrots, peeled and chopped

1 small onion, chopped

¼ cup chopped fresh mint

½ teaspoon ground ginger

½ teaspoon ground cumin

½ teaspoon ground turmeric

½ teaspoon paprika

½ teaspoon garlic powder

½ teaspoon red pepper flakes

⅛ teaspoon ground cinnamon

⅛ teaspoon ground coriander

⅛ teaspoon ground nutmeg

⅛ teaspoon ground cloves

Dash salt

Dash freshly ground black pepper

1. Pour the broth or water into the bottom of the slow cooker. Add the lamb, carrots, and onion.

2. In a small bowl, mix to combine the mint, ginger, cumin, turmeric, paprika, garlic powder, red pepper flakes, cinnamon, coriander, nutmeg, cloves, salt, and pepper. Sprinkle the mixture all over the lamb and vegetables, and stir to mix well.

3. Cook on low for 6 to 8 hours and serve.

COOKING TIP: Don't be surprised if you see a layer of melted lamb fat floating around in the slow cooker with this recipe. To remove it easily, let the dish cool first. Once cooled, you can scoop the fat off with a spoon.

PER SERVING Calories: 638; Total Fat: 48g; Saturated Fat: 22g; Cholesterol: 160mg; Sodium: 221mg; Potassium: 262mg; Carbs: 7g; Fiber: 3g; Protein: 39g

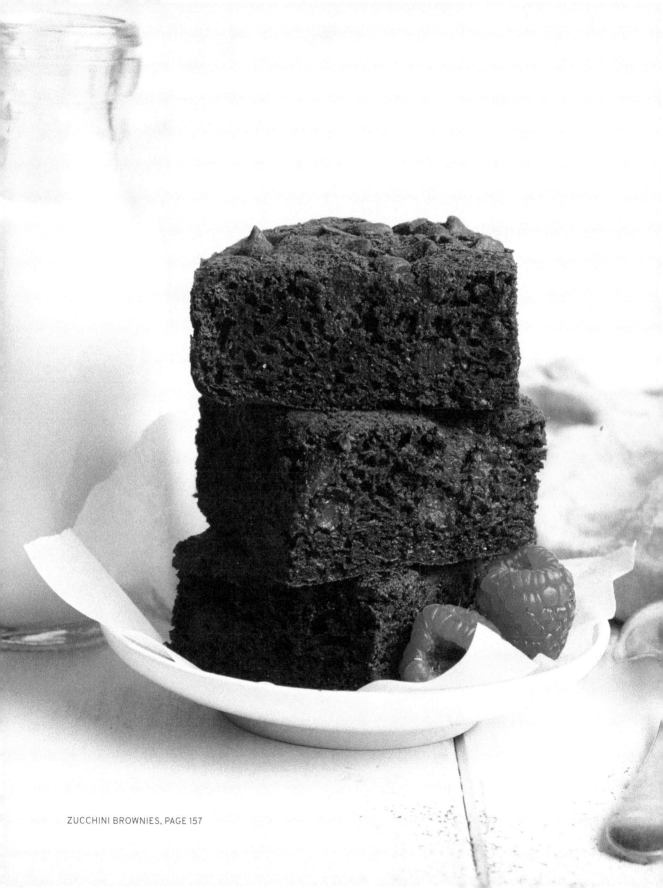

ZUCCHINI BROWNIES, PAGE 157

Desserts

Granola-Chocolate Bark

SERVES 8 • **PREP TIME:** 5 MINUTES, PLUS 15 MINUTES TO COOL
COOK TIME: 1 TO 3 HOURS ON LOW

LOWEST SODIUM

LOW-CHOLESTEROL • VEGETARIAN

This dessert is easy (only two ingredients!), but it's a sure hit. After breaking the bark into pieces, package it up and give it as gifts. You'll look like a master chef, and no one has to know how easy it was.

Nonstick cooking spray

1 pound Granola (page 36)

2 pounds semisweet chocolate chips

1. Spray the slow cooker generously with nonstick cooking spray.
2. Spread the granola evenly in the bottom of the slow cooker. Top with the chocolate chips.
3. Cook on low for 1 to 3 hours, or until the chocolate is completely melted.
4. Stir the chocolate and granola until thoroughly mixed.
5. Line a large baking sheet with parchment paper or aluminum foil. Transfer the mixture to the prepared baking sheet and spread in an even layer across the pan.
6. Let sit at room temperature to harden, or place in the refrigerator for 15 minutes.
7. Break or cut into about 36 pieces and serve.

VARIATION: Get creative with the add-ins. If your granola doesn't already include chopped nuts, seeds, or dried berries, add them at the start of cooking time.

PER SERVING Calories: 642; Total Fat: 37g; Saturated Fat: 21g; Cholesterol: 0mg; Sodium: 12mg; Potassium: 512mg; Carbs: 78g; Fiber: 8g; Protein: 6g

Sweet Granola Clusters

SERVES 6 • **PREP TIME:** 10 MINUTES • **COOK TIME:** 4 TO 6 HOURS ON LOW

LOWEST SODIUM

LOW-CHOLESTEROL • VEGETARIAN

Using healthy ingredients like oats, nuts, and honey, these granola clusters can be eaten for breakfast, post-workout, or as a quick snack on the go. I use natural ingredients, so you'll see that sugar is gone and honey or maple syrup is used in its place. These sweeteners don't cause a spike and then a crash in blood sugar the way processed sugar does.

Nonstick cooking spray

3 cups rolled oats

1 cup chopped nuts and seeds (almonds, pecans, walnuts, sunflower seeds, roasted pumpkin seeds, etc.)

¼ cup coconut oil, melted

⅔ cup honey (or maple syrup if vegan)

½ teaspoon pure vanilla extract

¼ teaspoon salt

1. Spray the slow cooker generously with nonstick cooking spray.
2. In the bottom of the slow cooker, mix to combine the oats, nuts, and seeds.
3. In a small bowl, mix together the coconut oil, honey, vanilla, and salt. Pour the mixture into the slow cooker, stirring to make sure all the ingredients are coated well.
4. Lay a dish towel or 2 paper towels between the slow cooker and the lid. This will absorb the condensation so it won't drip onto the crust while it cooks.
5. Cook on low for 4 to 6 hours.
6. Line a baking sheet with parchment paper or aluminum foil. Scoop the granola out of the cooker with a spoon, shape it into clusters or balls, and place on the parchment paper.
7. Cool to room temperature and serve.

INGREDIENT TIP: Oats are naturally gluten-free. They can cause a problem, though, when they are processed on equipment that also processes gluten grains, so make sure your oats are labeled gluten-free if that is an issue for you.

PER SERVING Calories: 623; Total Fat: 27g; Saturated Fat: 10g; Cholesterol: 0mg; Sodium: 100mg; Potassium: 440mg; Carbs: 85g; Fiber: 10g; Protein: 16g

Apple-Granola Bake

SERVES 6 • **PREP TIME:** 10 MINUTES • **COOK TIME:** 6 TO 8 HOURS ON LOW

LOW SODIUM

VEGETARIAN

I've placed this in the dessert chapter, but depending on your taste, you can have it for breakfast as well. You can use either steel-cut or rolled oats in this recipe without having to make any modifications.

Nonstick cooking spray

2 cups steel-cut oats

2 apples, finely diced, divided

⅓ cup semisweet chocolate chips, divided

1 teaspoon baking powder

1 teaspoon ground cinnamon

½ teaspoon salt

2 cups almond milk

¼ cup honey or maple syrup

1 ripe banana, mashed

1 large egg

1 tablespoon pure vanilla extract

1 banana, cut into ½-inch slices

1. Spray the slow cooker generously with nonstick cooking spray.

2. In a large bowl, mix together the oats, 1 of the diced apples, about half of the chocolate chips, and the baking powder, cinnamon, and salt.

3. In a separate large bowl, whisk together the almond milk, honey, mashed banana, egg, and vanilla. The honey might clump up at first; just keep whisking.

4. Pour the oat mixture into the slow cooker. Add the remaining apple and chocolate chips, and spread the banana slices on top.

5. Pour the honey mixture on top of everything. Gently shake the slow cooker to make sure all of the dry mixture is completely wet.

6. Cook on low for 6 to 8 hours, or until the oatmeal is set, and serve. (You'll know it's done when you insert a knife and it comes out clean.)

VARIATION: Berries like strawberries, blueberries, or raspberries work well instead of (or along with) apples.

PER SERVING Calories: 388; Total Fat: 8g; Saturated Fat: 3g; Cholesterol: 35mg; Sodium: 257mg; Potassium: 567mg; Carbs: 73g; Fiber: 9g; Protein: 11g

Zucchini Brownies

SERVES 8 • **PREP TIME:** 10 MINUTES • **COOK TIME:** 6 TO 8 HOURS ON LOW

LOW SODIUM

VEGETARIAN

Of course you can make brownies in the slow cooker! Adding zucchini makes them healthy and guiltless, too. This is a good recipe for incorporating whole-wheat flour, since the chocolate is the dominant flavor and can stand up to just about anything.

Nonstick cooking spray

2 large eggs

1 tablespoon pure vanilla extract

¾ cup coconut sugar or unrefined sugar

¼ cup Applesauce (page 34)

1 cup whole-wheat flour

½ cup unsweetened cocoa powder

1½ teaspoons baking soda

¼ teaspoon salt

2 cups peeled and grated zucchini

1 cup semisweet chocolate chips, divided

Cocoa powder, for dusting (optional)

1. Spray the slow cooker generously with nonstick cooking spray or line with parchment paper.
2. In a large bowl, mix together the eggs, vanilla, sugar, and applesauce.
3. In a medium bowl, mix together the flour, cocoa powder, baking soda, and salt.
4. Stir the dry ingredients into the wet ingredients until they're well combined. Gently fold in the zucchini and ½ cup of chocolate chips. Pour the mixture into the slow cooker.
5. Sprinkle the remaining ½ cup of chocolate chips on top.
6. Cook on low for 6 to 8 hours.
7. Remove from the slow cooker and cool completely before cutting into brownies. Dust with the cocoa powder (if using).

VARIATION: Add an extra ½ cup of chocolate chips on top of the brownies after they're done cooking, for garnish (and more chocolate!).

PER SERVING Calories: 234; Total Fat: 8g; Saturated Fat: 5g; Cholesterol: 53mg; Sodium: 327mg; Potassium: 289mg; Carbs: 40g; Fiber: 5g; Protein: 5g

Peach Crumble

SERVES 4 • **PREP TIME:** 10 MINUTES • **COOK TIME:** 2 TO 3 HOURS ON LOW

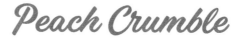

LOW-CHOLESTEROL • VEGETARIAN

This dessert couldn't get any easier; it's just peaches and granola. If you like your crumble a little sweeter, try adding a natural sweetener like honey or maple syrup. Depending on what type of granola you use or how sweet your fruit is, you might not need any. This doesn't have to be a peach crumble, either. Make it a berry one. The variations are endless. You can use whatever combo of fruits you please.

Nonstick cooking spray

6 cups peaches, pitted and sliced

2 cups Granola (page 36)

1. Spray the slow cooker generously with nonstick cooking spray.

2. Put the peaches in the bottom of the slow cooker, and spread the granola on top.

3. Lay a small towel or 2 paper towels in between the slow cooker and the lid to create a barrier. This will catch all the condensation so it won't drip onto the granola while it cooks.

4. Cook on low for 2 to 3 hours, or until the peaches are bubbling.

INGREDIENT TIP: Fresh fruit can be expensive when it's out of season—and not especially flavorful. Frozen fruit is perfectly fine to use. It's not only cheaper and available year-round, but the nutrients and fiber are still there.

PER SERVING Calories: 290; Total Fat: 7g; Saturated Fat: 3g; Cholesterol: 0mg; Sodium: 1mg; Potassium: 607mg; Carbs: 53g; Fiber: 8g; Protein: 8g

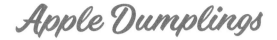

Apple Dumplings

MAKES 16 • **PREP TIME:** 10 MINUTES • **COOK TIME:** 2 TO 4 HOURS ON LOW

LOWER SODIUM

LOW-CARB • LOW-CHOLESTEROL • VEGETARIAN

This recipe uses store-bought low-fat crescent rolls—the kind that come in a tube. Low-fat and organic versions of these pop-can rolls are relatively new. There's even a commercial gluten-free pizza dough that comes in a tub and would work just fine for this recipe, if gluten is an issue for you.

Nonstick cooking spray

2 apples, peeled, cored, and sliced

2 packages low-fat crescent rolls

¼ cup Applesauce (page 34)

4 tablespoons unsalted butter, melted

½ cup honey

2 teaspoons ground cinnamon

1. Spray your slow cooker generously with nonstick cooking spray.

2. Take one slice of apple and wrap one crescent roll around the apple slice, starting with the small end of the crescent roll. Repeat with the remaining slices and rolls. Place the wrapped slices in the bottom of the slow cooker.

3. In a small bowl, mix together the applesauce, butter, honey, and cinnamon. Pour the mixture on top of all your dumplings.

4. Cook on low for 2 to 4 hours and serve.

SUBSTITUTION TIP: Use maple syrup and coconut oil instead of honey and butter to make this a vegan dessert.

PER SERVING (4 PIECES) Calories: 159; Total Fat: 6g; Saturated Fat: 3g; Cholesterol: 8mg; Sodium: 221mg; Potassium: 31mg; Carbs: 25g; Fiber: 1g; Protein: 2g

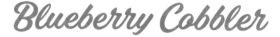

Blueberry Cobbler

SERVES 4 • **PREP TIME:** 15 MINUTES • **COOK TIME:** 4 TO 5 HOURS ON LOW

LOWER SODIUM

GLUTEN-FREE • LOW-CHOLESTEROL • VEGETARIAN

This recipe uses oat flour. Oats are a good source of fiber and antioxidants. Making your own oat flour is easy. All you do is put your rolled oats in a food processor and grind until they reach your desired flour consistency.

6 cups blueberries

¼ cup Fruit Jam (page 33)

⅓ cup honey or maple syrup plus 2 tablespoons, divided

2 teaspoons pure vanilla extract, divided

1½ cups rolled oats, ground to flour

2 to 3 tablespoons almond milk

1 teaspoon baking powder

1 teaspoon ground cinnamon

¼ teaspoon salt

Nonstick cooking spray

1 tablespoon butter or ghee (clarified butter)

1. In a large bowl, combine the blueberries, fruit jam, ⅓ cup of honey, and 1 teaspoon of vanilla. Stir to combine well. Set aside.

2. In a medium bowl, whisk together the oat flour, the remaining 2 tablespoons of honey, and the almond milk, baking powder, cinnamon, the remaining 1 teaspoon of vanilla, and the salt to make the cobbler.

3. Lightly spray the bottom of the slow cooker with non-stick cooking spray. Crumble the cobbler evenly over the bottom of the slow cooker, and pour the fruit on top. Spread dollops of butter evenly over the fruit.

4. Cook on low for 4 to 5 hours, or until the blueberries are bubbling, cool slightly, and serve.

VARIATION: While this is blueberry cobbler, you can swap the blueberries for diced peaches or another fruit. Fresh or frozen fruit will be fine here.

PER SERVING Calories: 526; Total Fat: 5g; Saturated Fat: 1g; Cholesterol: 0mg; Sodium: 158mg; Potassium: 583mg; Carbs: 116g; Fiber: 12g; Protein: 12g

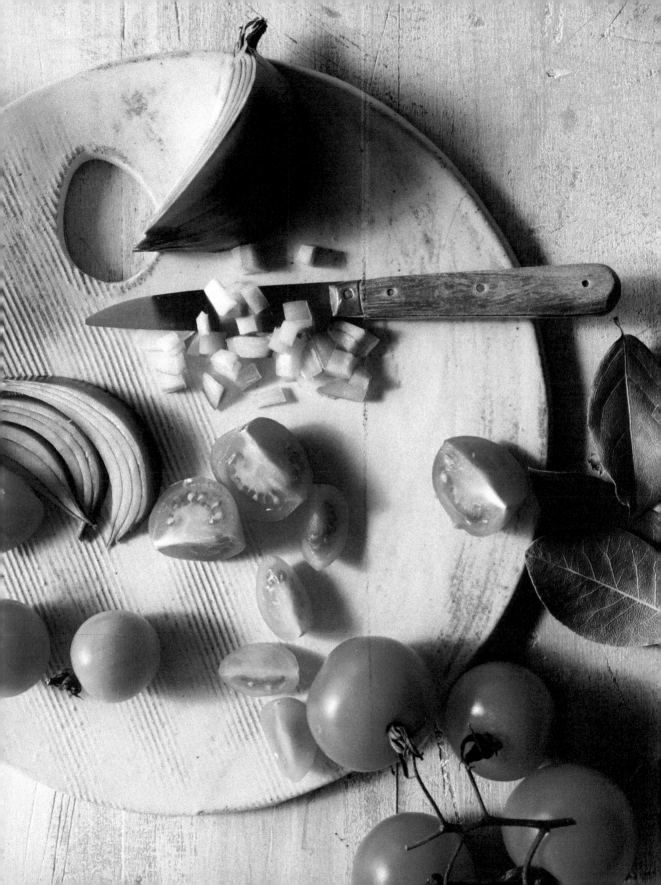

APPENDIX A
Tips for Eating Out

YOU'VE PUT IN ALL THIS HARD WORK WITH A HEALTHY, LOW-SODIUM lifestyle, and now it's time to eat out. Don't be scared. It's possible to eat out without derailing your low-sodium diet. Here are a few tips to keep yourself on track:

- **Ask for a modification.** It sounds simple because it is. Most restaurants will take a special request, particularly when it's dietary. Simply asking for dressing on the side, no sauce, or even asking that no salt be added to your food can make a big difference in your sodium intake. Yes, there will still be some sodium in the food, but you can at least avoid any extra added in. You have to choose your food wisely, of course. Asking for no salt on a pizza doesn't make much of a difference. (Speaking of pizzas, they're not the best option when eating out. Pizza, cheese, cured meats, breads, and soups all tend to have higher sodium levels, so it's best to limit these types of foods.)

- **No frying.** Whether we're talking about meat or vegetables, order your food baked, broiled, grilled, roasted, or steamed. Avoid fried food at all costs.

- **Limit sauces and condiments.** Most sauces and condiments contribute a lot of sodium. Ketchup and salsa, in particular, are low-calorie but tend to have higher sodium levels.

- **Skip the chips.** Tell them not to bring chips to your table the moment you sit down. If they bring chips and salsa to the table, immediately ask them to take it away. Also beware of pickles and olives, which are cured in salty brine.

- **Choose wisely.** Stay away from restaurants you know will throw you off track. Try to eat at restaurants known to cook their food to order. Local restaurants are good options for this. Big restaurant chains aren't necessarily bad; some provide nutritional information on their menus now.

- **Control your sides.** Main dishes can be a little tricky, but sides are usually simpler. Order your vegetables steamed. Vegetables are not only healthy but naturally low in sodium. Ask for no salt and add a sprinkle yourself at the table.
- **Skip dessert.** How about fruit instead? If the restaurant doesn't have fruit, how about sorbet?
- **Taste your food.** Sounds silly, but I mean this. Taste the food when it comes. Is it too salty? Send it back. Your health is worth being finicky. Especially taste the food before *adding* any salt or condiments.

Measurement Conversions

VOLUME EQUIVALENTS (LIQUID)

US STANDARD	US STANDARD (OUNCES)	METRIC (APPROXIMATE)
2 tablespoons	1 fl. oz.	30 mL
¼ cup	2 fl. oz.	60 mL
½ cup	4 fl. oz.	120 mL
1 cup	8 fl. oz.	240 mL
1½ cups	12 fl. oz.	355 mL
2 cups or 1 pint	16 fl. oz.	475 mL
4 cups or 1 quart	32 fl. oz.	1 L
1 gallon	128 fl. oz.	4 L

OVEN TEMPERATURES

FAHRENHEIT	CELSIUS (APPROXIMATE)
250°F	120°C
300°F	150°C
325°F	165°C
350°F	180°C
375°F	190°C
400°F	200°C
425°F	220°C
450°F	230°C

VOLUME EQUIVALENTS (DRY)

US STANDARD	METRIC (APPROXIMATE)
⅛ teaspoon	0.5 mL
¼ teaspoon	1 mL
½ teaspoon	2 mL
¾ teaspoon	4 mL
1 teaspoon	5 mL
1 tablespoon	15 mL
¼ cup	59 mL
⅓ cup	79 mL
½ cup	118 mL
⅔ cup	156 mL
¾ cup	177 mL
1 cup	235 mL
2 cups or 1 pint	475 mL
3 cups	700 mL
4 cups or 1 quart	1 L

WEIGHT EQUIVALENTS

US STANDARD	METRIC (APPROXIMATE)
½ ounce	15 g
1 ounce	30 g
2 ounces	60 g
4 ounces	115 g
8 ounces	225 g
12 ounces	340 g
16 ounces or 1 pound	455 g

The Dirty Dozen and the Clean Fifteen™

A nonprofit environmental watchdog organization called Environmental Working Group (EWG) looks at data supplied by the US Department of Agriculture (USDA) and the Food and Drug Administration (FDA) about pesticide residues. Each year it compiles a list of the best and worst pesticide loads found in commercial crops. You can use these lists to decide which fruits and vegetables to buy organic to minimize your exposure to pesticides and which produce is considered safe enough to buy conventionally. This does not mean they are pesticide-free, though, so wash these fruits and vegetables thoroughly.

These lists change every year, so make sure you look up the most recent one before you fill your shopping cart. You'll find the most recent lists, as well as a guide to pesticides in produce, at EWG.org/FoodNews.

DIRTY DOZEN

Apples
Celery
Cherries
Cherry tomatoes
Cucumbers
Grapes
Nectarines
Peaches
Spinach
Strawberries
Sweet bell peppers
Tomatoes

In addition to the Dirty Dozen, the EWG added two types of produce contaminated with highly toxic organophosphate insecticides:

Kale/Collard greens
Hot peppers

CLEAN FIFTEEN

Asparagus
Avocados
Cabbage
Cantaloupe
Cauliflower
Eggplant
Grapefruit
Honeydew melon

Kiwifruits
Mangos
Onions
Papayas
Pineapples
Sweet corn
Sweet peas (frozen)

Recipe Index

Index

M

Acknowledgments

Thank you to my husband, Lawrence, for your constant support and for encouraging me to reach for my dreams. To my parents, father-in-law, siblings, family, and friends all over the world—I love you all. Your support means so much. To all of my followers, on my blog and on social media, I seriously wouldn't be here without you. I'm so grateful you're out there. Finally, to Callisto Media, in particular Elizabeth Castoria for bringing another opportunity to my plate and Nana K. Twumasi for being so patient and kind. You have helped to make this experience a pleasure.

About the Author

SHANNON EPSTEIN is a full-time food and travel writer. She is the author of *The Easy and Healthy Slow Cooker Cookbook* and has two blogs, FitSlowCookerQueen.com (healthy slow cooker recipes) and TweetEatTravel.com (travel and lifestyle). Shannon lives in Los Angeles with her husband.

Printed in the USA
CPSIA information can be obtained
at www.ICGtesting.com
LVHW051929091223
765801LV00003B/20